THE EIGHT
EXTRAORDINARY
MERIDIANS

MONKEY PRESS
Monkey Press is named after the Monkey King in The Journey to the West, the 16th century novel by Wu Chengen. Monkey blends skill, initiative and wisdom with the spirit of freedom, irreverence and a touch of mischief.

CHINESE MEDICINE FROM THE CLASSICS

Claude Larre and Elisabeth Rochat de la Vallée:
The Secret Treatise of the Spiritual Orchid
The Lung
The Kidneys
The Heart in Lingshu chapter 8
Heart Master Triple Heater
The Liver
Spleen and Stomach
The Way of Heaven
Essence Spirit Blood and Qi
The Seven Emotions
The Extraordinary Fu

Elisabeth Rochat de la Vallée:
A Study of Qi
Yin Yang in Classical Texts
The Essential Woman
Pregnancy and Gestation
Wu Xing: The Five Elements
The Rhythm at the Heart of the World: Suwen chapter 5
The Double Aspect of the Heart
Aspects of Spirit

Group translation:
Jing Shen: Huainanzi chapter 7

Sandra Hill:
Chinese Medicine from the Classics: a beginner's guide

THE EIGHT
EXTRAORDINARY MERIDIANS

Claude Larre and Elisabeth Rochat de la Vallée

transcribed and edited by Sandra Hill

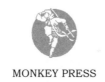

MONKEY PRESS

Published by
Monkey Press
www.monkeypress.net
info@monkeypress.net

CHINESE MEDICINE FROM THE CLASSICS:
THE EIGHT EXTRAORDINARY MERIDIANS
Claude Larre and Elisabeth Rochat de la Vallée

ISBN 978 1 872468 13 6

Text editor: Sandra Hill
Calligraphy: Qu Lei Lei
Printed in the UK by Short Run Press

奇經八脈

CONTENTS

FOREWORD

The work of sinologists Claude Larre and Elisabeth Rochat de la Vallée gives us access to the classical origins of Chinese medicine. Through Claude Larre's profound understanding of the philosophical and cultural background, and Elisabeth Rochat's thorough knowledge of the classical medical texts we are able to gain a unique insight into the mysterious nature of these eight extraordinary meridians. Close examination of the original texts of the Neijing, Nanjing and their commentaries, provides a detailed analysis of their functions, pathways and pathologies.

The text has been edited from two three day seminars and retains some of the conversational style of the original teachings. It is not intended as an historical overview, nor as a guide to a specific mode of practice – throughout the long history of Chinese medicine, this subject has been presented in many different ways by many different schools. Through study of the classical texts we discover that this primitive organization into eight meridians governs the relationships between *yin* and *yang*, interior and exterior, providing the basic patterning for the development and maintenance of the body. They provide the foundation for the division into the more accessible twelve ordinary meridians.

When recently teaching a class of first year acupuncture students I was reminded of the usual status given to this subject – a few pages at the back of a text book, or an afternoon tacked on the end of a crowded syllabus. These eight meridians are often seen simply as something 'extra', almost superfluous, rather than the extraordinary and 'marvellous' foundation of our entire energetic network. It is my hope that this book goes some way to redress that balance.

Sandra Hill
London, 1997

Foreword to the second edition:

During the considerable time that has elapsed since its first printing, this book has not diminished in importance; it remains the only study of the eight extraordinary meridians from the texts of the Neijing and Nanjing. Its elucidation of texts from these two sources provide an invaluable insight into the use of these channels in both acupuncture practice and inner cultivation.

This second edition of the text contains minor changes, some clarification and updates of the terminology, but the translation of the Chinese aims to remain true to the original text, and does not always follow modern convention when this is considered inappropriate to convey classical meaning. Claude and Elisabeth often refer in the text to 'Chinese Characters' by Dr. L. Wieger (Dover Publications) which is a translation based on the 2nd century CE etymological dictionary the Shuowen Jiezi.

Sandra Hill
London, 2015

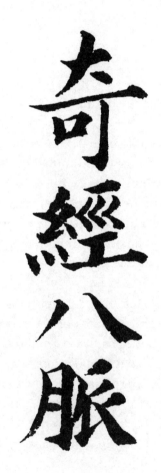

qi jing ba mai

INTRODUCTION

Claude Larre: Our subject is the extraordinary meridians, the *qi jing ba mai* (奇 經 八 脈), which are not only extraordinary, but marvellous. I personally prefer to use the word extraordinary, but there is also this other aspect – that they are doing marvels. Perhaps they are extraordinary because they are part of the primitive constitution of the being, and represent the purest stimulation of life given by heaven, which is in itself an extraordinary power when contrasted with earth, where things are developed and seen. Heaven represents the creation of life and the invisible power of life. So when something is unseen but working for life, it has the attribute of being a truly marvellous thing.

For that reason the *qi jing ba mai* must be seen as the foundation of life from its very beginning to its very end. They are active from conception to birth, working within a state of life which is not fully organized. With the development of the arms and legs, hands and feet, the number twelve is appropriate and comes into full effect after birth; but the twelve ordinary meridians take their strength from the origin of life. The number twelve is the natural extension of four (of the four limbs) stimulated by the power of the *qi* which is represented by the number three. So in the developed form of a human being, heaven and earth work through twelve different pathways, and in contrast to that, the more primitive form is like winds in the atmosphere. The winds are governed by the number eight, which is four times two, and these eight winds provide the general movement of the universe.

This distinction between the twelve which are ordinary and the eight which are extraordinary is very appropriate – not just for the beginning but also for the end of life. Because the beginning and the end of life have to turn, or return, in a circle. When the meridians become eight from twelve, that could signify the return of that person to a previous state of life, no longer governed by the feet and the hands. The feet and hands stop their activity, the power of the person is absorbed and there is no longer a way to manifest externally. That seed of life has to be there at the end of life as it has been at the beginning. So the Chinese expression *qi jing ba mai*, the eight extraordinary meridians, is a very good one.

Elisabeth Rochat: This expression appears for the first time in Nanjing difficulty 27, and as Father Larre has said, it is a very good expression to describe these eight extraordinary meridians. The extraordinary meridians do not appear as a complete set in the Suwen or Lingshu. In one chapter there is a reference to the *ren mai* and *chong mai*, in another chapter *chong mai* with the kidney meridian, in another a mention of the *qiao mai* etc., but it is in the Nanjing that they are organized and gathered together for the first time in written form, though they might have existed before as oral teachings or in lost texts.

STUDY OF THE CHARACTERS

Elisabeth Rochat: In the name *qi jing ba mai* (奇 經 八 脈) each character is important. As usual in Chinese we begin with the end.

MAI 脈
Mai (脈) is a general word for the vital circulation, meridians (*jing* 經), as well as *luo* (絡) and all other kinds of circulation. There are *mai* in the depths and there are *mai* up to the surface of the body. The *qi jing ba mai* are the expression of this general network of animation as expressed by the number eight.

BA 八
As Father Larre has said, eight (*ba* 八) is very important because it is the number of the winds and the distribution of vitality, essences and spirit. In the depths of our being we have five *zang* and six *fu*. The number seven then represents a kind of bursting out of vitality, which is why there are seven upper orifices, and seven emotions – seven is the number related to this spreading of vitality. Eight is the appropriate number for the penetration of all space by the vitality coming from seven. Through the symbolism of numerology and graphology, there is a kind of division, an initial differentiation. We move from the area of undifferentiated *qi* to a network of vital circulation, which occupies space in order to distribute spirits, essences and *qi*.

JING 經

These eight are not only *mai* (脈) but also *jing* (經) or meridians. A meridian is a norm. It is a basic principle for the organization and vital circulation of life, which relies on the model and principle of heaven, but which also takes into account the earthly surroundings and the earthly shape of the body. This is the meaning of *jing*. There are only twelve *jing*, only twelve meridians, and it is important to understand that the *luo* (絡) or the *bie* (別), the so-called divergent meridians, are not *jing*, and they are not called meridians in the Chinese.

The texts tell us that there are only twelve meridians, but now these eight are also called meridians, and at the symbolic level of eight they represent the organization of the territory inside the body and control all the powers of life which create the human body and keep it in balance. They allow the manifestation of the great principle of cosmic balance within the body, but do not have a relationship with the external surroundings. These eight extraordinary meridians do not exactly divide the bodily territory or area into eight parts as do the twelve ordinary meridians. Generally speaking, they share pathways and their pathways may have common origins, as for example with *du mai* (督脈 governor vessel), *ren mai* (任脈 conception vessel) and *chong mai* (衝脈 penetrating vessel), while this kind of sharing of pathways does not happen at all with the twelve ordinary meridians. We can see that the separation is much more clear cut for the twelve meridians than for the eight extraordinary meridians. So, although they are also called meridians, they do not have the same purpose. They are rather for the inner organization of life and prepare the way for the twelve meridians within the adult, which just influence their own areas, but are also able to resonate and respond to external influences. That is why these meridians are called *qi* (奇), extraordinary, marvellous, singular, and so on – and this character has a lot of very interesting meanings.

QI 奇

Qi (奇) is extraordinary, surprising and strange, and etymologically speaking it is a human being uttering an exclamation of surprise. But *qi* (奇) can also mean marvellous – so marvellous that it is beyond compare, utterly unique. With the meaning of unique we also understand single and odd, like the odd numbers which are single and unique because they are not divisible by two. Another meaning can be irregular, against the norm, because if you are unique you are very close to being an anarchist.

Another important classical meaning is of a kind of fraction, the remainder of a fraction in division, or the small remainder when time or space are cut geometrically. For instance, the day has twelve or 24 hours which is very efficient and useful for our watches and our schedules, but astronomically speaking it is not quite accurate, there are always some seconds remaining. In Chinese this is called *qi* (奇). It is the same for the year; there are 365 days but it is not exact, and this remainder is also *qi* (奇).

These meridians are singular and extraordinary, because they are different from the other meridians which are called *zheng* (正), correct, ordinary, without any diversion. The extraordinary meridians are not so tied by principles, not so constrained and constricted. The twelve ordinary meridians relate to each other in couples in a face/interface, internal/external, *biao/li* (表 理) relationship and they make couples as foot and hand meridians. They also have a special relationship with the *zangfu*, each meridian having its specific *zang* or *fu*. These normal meridians also have a correspondence to the five elements through the *zangfu*, and through the external heavenly influxes, cold, heat, wind, damp, dryness and fire, and according to Lingshu chapter 12 they have a special correspondence with the rivers on earth:

> '...the *jing mai* relate on the exterior to the twelve water courses, and on the interior are under the authority of the five *zang* and the six *fu*.'

The *qi jing ba mai* have none of that, they have no paired relationships, and in that way they are also strange and extraordinary. Some relationships are mentioned in later texts, for example between *du mai* and *yang qiao mai*, but it was much later, and it has nothing to do with the *biao/li*, face/interface relationship, it has another meaning. These eight meridians also have no hand and foot differentiation, they hardly appear in the legs and not at all on the arms. As far as *du mai*, *ren mai*, *chong mai* and *dai mai* are concerned, there is no quality of *yin* and *yang* in their names. There is no special relationship with the *zang* and *fu*: not that they have no relationships to the *zang* and *fu*, but these relationships are not regular and systematic. There is not a relationship between one extraordinary meridian and one *zang* or one *fu*, but rather the extraordinary meridians represent the original organization of the *yin*, and the original organization of the *yang* everywhere in the body.

With the twelve meridians there is always the relationship with the elements, the months of the year or with external influences, as we see in Lingshu chapter 11:

> 'The twelve meridians themselves unite with the twelve months and the twelve constellations and the twelve articulations of animation (*jie* 節), the twelve watercourses, the twelve double hours of the day, the vital circulation of the twelve meridians.'

It is through the animating network of the twelve ordinary meridians that human beings live, interact and that illnesses manifest themselves. It is through the twelve that we treat illness. All study begins with them and all working ends with them, because the acupuncture points are only on the twelve meridians, *du mai* and *ren mai* – the other extraordinary meridians have no points of their own. If these meridians are so strange and they are not in correspondence and resonance with the elements, the seasons and the external influx, how can they be meridians or 'norms' for the vital circulation? If we look at the texts of the Nanjing we can see that there are some kind of special correspondences.

NANJING difficulty 27

The first presentation and explanation is given in Nanjing difficulty 27.

'The *mai* include the *qi jing ba mai*, the eight *mai* of the extraordinary meridians, eight *mai* which are not linked with the twelve meridians. What can one say of them?

'Well, there are the *yang wei* (陽 維), there are the *yin wei* (陰 維). There are the *yang qiao* (陽 蹻), there are the *yin qiao* (陰 蹻); there is the *chong* (衝), there is the *du* (督), there is the *dai* (帶) there is the *ren* (任). That is to say there are eight *mai* which are not connected to the twelve meridians. It is because of this that one talks of the *qi jing ba mai*. The meridians are twelve, the *luo* are 15; in all that makes 27 *qi*, they follow each other, rising and falling.

'Why are these not included in the meridians?

'Well, the scheme for the saintly man (*sheng ren* 聖 人) lays out canals and channels (*gou qu* 溝 渠) for the easy circulation (*tong* 通) of the waterways (*shui dao* 水 道); this is to guard against unexpected circumstances. When rain descends from heaven, canals and channels fill up to create rambling (overflow, *wang xing* 妄 行), then at the moment the saintly man can no longer turn to his ordinary scheme the *luo mai* are full up and overflow. This is why the twelve meridians cannot be the system of reference for the extraordinary meridians.'

This is the text that has given the idea that the eight extraordinary meridians act as some kind of reservoir for the ordinary meridians when they overflow. It is also the origin of the theory that the extraordinary meridians do not exist except when there is a fullness of the ordinary meridians. But that is not in the Chinese text. That is not exactly the meaning of this difficulty of the Nanjing and it is certainly not possible in context of all the other Chinese texts, especially the Neijing. It is impossible to say that the extraordinary meridians only exist when the overflowing of the ordinary meridians demands it, because there are descriptions of them independent of this kind of fullness, where they have their own functions and responsibilities. For instance in Suwen chapter 1 the *ren mai* and *chong mai* are responsible for fertility in women, and there is no question of an overflow from the main meridians. And if the *qiao mai* are responsible for the circulation of defensive *qi*, and for the alternation of sleeping and waking during night and day, they are always functioning.

But this text is very interesting. Why are these eight *mai* not linked with the twelve meridians; why are they not the same as the twelve meridians? The answer is that they do not have the same paired relationship between inside and outside as the twelve meridians. They really are different, which is another meaning of *qi* (奇).

So what exactly is the meaning of these 'canals and ditches' which allow good circulation of the waterways? I think that it is a representation in the body of the organization of territory by the pattern of the waterways, such as was done by Yu the Great – because the organization of life, whether on the earth or within the body, obeys the same general rules. There is really no difference. If you take care of all the ditches and canals and channels you can avoid overflowing or flooding, so this is a way to provide protection. The extraordinary meridians are like ditches between great rivers, and in the body they have the function of passages and openings between the twelve or twenty four ordinary meridians. They provide a way to take preventive measures against unforeseen circumstances.

But is this the only meaning, that they are like reservoirs, full with an unexpected arrival of something like rain, causing an overflow of water on earth? I think that is just an image. The meaning is that because these meridians are older, more ancient than the ordinary meridians, when extraordinary circumstances exist outside, and the twelve main meridians can no longer ensure the maintenance of the twelve areas of the body, there is a return to a more ancient and deeper regulation of life. Here we have one of the meanings of these extraordinary meridians and of their role: it is to preserve the norm, but at a deeper level.

Suwen chapter 2 gives us a presentation of the four seasons. The first part of this chapter is the presentation of spring, summer, autumn and winter, the qualities proper to each of these seasons and the appropriate conduct to adopt and follow in order to respond to the season and be in good health. But the second part of the chapter gives an example of extraordinary, unforeseeable circumstances, very bad weather – hurricanes, tornadoes, very heavy rain, or drought

– the kind of circumstances which endanger all living beings. In this case, the saint of the text is able to regulate his vital circulation, and this is the reason why he has no extraordinary illness. This is the same word 'extraordinary' (*qi* 奇) and in this context the meaning is that this extraordinary illness came about through very strange and unusual circumstances. An ordinary person who is unable to return to something deeper than the twelve meridians to organize life, is unable to cope with these circumstances and to resist the effect of the environmental extremes. This is one way in which the extraordinary meridians regulate in the depths, because they are the last resort, or the deepest resort, like a kind of prototype of the whole organization and the relationships that take place in the unfolding of the body.

We can find the same opposition, which is at the same time complementary, between what is *zheng* (正), correct or ordinary or usual, and *qi* (奇), extraordinary. In books on military strategy, especially The Art of War, *zheng* (正) designates the usual armed forces, and *qi* (奇) designates something which is not within the normal or usual principles of battle. This *qi* can refer to all kinds of unexpected movements of troops, such as suddenly coming from behind, with the effect of a surprise attack. The Art of War says that if the enemy sees that an operation is an extraordinary operation, it then becomes an ordinary operation, because the element of surprise is lost. Sunzi also says that while you can begin the battle with ordinary forces, you can be victorious only with the use of extraordinary forces. This is not a case of opposition, but a perpetual movement between that which is ordinary and that which is extraordinary in order to win the battle – one supports the other. To win the battle on the battlefield is the same as winning the battle of life: to remain in the best state of health and life. And we have to use both at the same time, the extraordinary being the invisible part of the ordinary, as it is in battle. It is not exactly the same in the body, but it is useful to draw comparisons.

The final meaning of *qi* (奇) as a kind of remainder of a fraction, a little space of time which is the remainder of the day or the year, is seen, for example, in Lingshu chapter 76. It describes the circulation of the defensive *qi*, and because time is divided very strictly into divisions of 14 minutes there is a unity of time, and the defensive *qi* has a particular movement. But because this strict outline of time and the length of all the pathways of circulation within the body do not completely correspond, there is a little difference between the external measure of time and the circulation of the defensive *qi*. This is called *qi* (奇).

In Suwen chapter 9 there is the same thing, but with the calendar. If we do not use an intercalary month, we will find that everything eventually goes out of sync. The Chinese used the double system of the solar and lunar calendar. Some parts of the measurement of time were made by the sun, others with the moon. After a while the difference between them was very apparent and would create problems with agriculture. With this *qi*, this fraction of time, they introduced an intercalary month every three or five years depending on the particular dynasty.

So what does this mean in the context of the extraordinary

meridians? They provide a way to regulate all kinds of cycles at a deeper level. Most systems of regulation are so just and exact that they are false. It is easier to have 24 hours in a day, but reality is not quite like that. This *qi* gives us the ability to readjust to a deeper reality, the most primitive reality of life, which lies behind that which is regulated by the seasons and correspondences and so on, which belong to the twelve.

The best way to interpret Nanjing difficulty 27 is to see the rain as an example of the regulation of waterways on earth. Waterways (*shui dao* 水 道) are a common metaphor for the *qi* (氣) and the circulation of *qi* in the body. The overflowing of the *luo mai* (絡 脈), the ordinary network of meridians, is a result of the inability to readjust, because the cycles are too regular and too limited by their regularity, and perhaps because outside circumstances are too powerful.

Claude Larre: It is like the difference between the harmony of music and the harmony of acoustic. If you were to rely on the acoustic to tune your piano or anything else, you would miss the point each time. So you ask someone who has a good ear with perfect hearing, and they may make a very small adjustment to the acoustic, but they are tuning to perfection. This is the same thing. The regulation of the twelve can be corrected through the system of the eight, which is more permissive, it allows more room for adjustment.

Question: When you mentioned that it was more primitive do you mean preceding in time?

Elisabeth Rochat: I think it also suggests that, yes. There is no Chinese text that says it exactly, but the eight are beneath and behind the twelve meridians. For example, *chong mai* is behind both the kidney and stomach meridians. And the explanation is either that it is the emanation of both these meridians or that both the kidney and stomach meridians are a double emanation of all the richness of *chong mai*. In this case there is a process of differentiation from the extraordinary meridians to the twelve meridians. It is more confused at the level of the extraordinary meridians in the sense that everything is more mixed together, less differentiated. Look, for example, at the common origin of the *chong mai*, *du mai* and *ren mai*. They are in that sense undifferentiated. The three are together at the origin, and then they begin to be differentiated, like the first divergence into three branches. It is a kind of territorial construction, but there is definitely something primitive, even in time, in the extraordinary meridians.

The twelve ordinary meridians are for the circulation of the blood and *qi*, as we see in Nanjing difficulty 23:

> '...the *jingmai* circulate blood and *qi*, they ensure free communication of *yinyang* so that the body can flourish.'

The extraordinary meridians ensure the regulation and the first laws for the relationship and circulation of blood and *qi*, essences and *qi*, and *yin* and *yang*. Blood circulation is originally regulated by *ren mai* and *chong mai*, but when the functions of the body are more clearly differentiated, the meridians and *zangfu*, for example the liver, kidneys and heart, take this circulation of blood under their authority. The liver meridian is important, for instance, because the circulation of blood refers not only to a good circulation through the blood vessels, but also to menstruation in a woman, and all kinds of particularities of the blood in a man, for example to enable the beard to grow, as we see in the Lingshu.

All these inner regulations are the cause of many problems in the life of a human being, and it is this first structuring of the regulation of blood and *qi* within the body which is the task of the extraordinary meridians. *Du mai* can be seen as the first elaboration of *qi* and *yang* in the body and *ren mai* as the first elaboration and structuring of the blood and *yin*. In this way *du mai* is not just a meridian on the back of the body, but, as we shall see, it has a more complex pathway and trajectory.

Du mai is the tension of all the *yang qi* in the body and *ren mai* brings together within the whole body the blood and the *yin* and the fluids. *Chong mai* is like an harmonious conjunction of both and a bursting out of vitality. In each living being there is always a conjunction of opposition of the two aspects of reality, *yin* and *yang*, water and fire, blood and *qi* and so on, and *chong mai* sums it all up in a kind of unity, which is the reason why we see it as a great motivator of life. *Dai mai* encloses the space of a living being within its natural boundaries, which gives us the beginning of a framework, a container – which contains and conducts at the same time.

Yin and *yang qiao mai* are the interpenetration and rhythm between *yin* and *yang*, and *yin* and *yang wei mai* are the inner organization of each system, the *yang* and *qi* and the *yin* and blood; they maintain the particular cohesion in each system. After this framework is established, all the more complicated relationships can take place through the complete system of the twelve meridians. According to Li Zhongzi:

> '...The *yang wei* has a special mastery over the exterior, *biao* (表). The *yin wei* on the interior, *li* (理).'

The *yang wei* and *yin wei mai* are often related to the two trigrams *qian* and *kun* – *qian* being the trigram representing the powerful effects of heaven, and *kun* those of earth. We will not go into depth about the relationship between the eight extraordinary meridians and the trigrams, and in some texts *yang wei* and *yin wei* may be related to other trigrams.

> '...*Yang qiao* has a special mastery over the *yang* on the left and right side of the body and the *yin qiao* a special mastery of the *yin* on the left and right side of the body.'

This is in order to indicate order, rhythm and inter-relationship and is the reason why the *yang qiao* corresponds to the east, and *yin qiao* to the west. Also, because rising movement occurs on the left and descending movement on the right, east is on the left, and west on the right, in accordance with the movement of the sun.

> '...*Du mai* has mastery over the *yang* at the rear of the

body, and the *ren mai* over the *yin* at the front. This is why they are south and north.

'*Dai mai* is like an horizontal link tying together all the network of vital circulation, and it corresponds to the six junctions, *liu he* (六 合).'

In this text there is no mention of *chong mai*. I think it is because it is like the connection of the power of *du mai* and *ren mai*. Li Shizhen, who wrote a special study on the extraordinary meridians, related *chong mai* with *du mai* and *ren mai*. There is no coupled relationship of *dai mai* and *chong mai*.

But what is the explanation of this strange presentation? The six junctions are the vital space between heaven and earth, the first exchanges of *qi* which define the territory within which livings being appear. This fits quite well with the idea of *dai mai*. Here we have the four directions: south and north, the great axis for rising up and descending, the vertical axis between heaven and earth, and the horizontal axis, east and west, with all kinds of exchanges in daily life between left and right, *yin* and *yang*, male and female, interior and exterior. All this is influenced by the *qiao mai* and the *wei mai*.

When the classical Chinese authors make a comparison between the extraordinary meridians and something in nature, they do not use the elements or rivers or seasons or *qi* coming from heaven, they use the first division of space, the first junction between heaven and earth, the first framework of organization of space, in the form of the four directions, and the two first trigrams which express the appearance of the forces of nature at the origin of life. They take the extraordinary meridians and couple them with the most basic and primitive orientations of life, putting the living being in the right place within the universe, rather than making point by point correspondences.

Claude Larre: Within any Chinese text it is usual to start with *tian di* (天 地), heaven and earth, and *si shi* (四 時), four seasons. When the Chinese speak of heaven and earth they are saying that the play of life is between the creative and the receptive. The expressions creative and receptive are used in the Book of Changes because heaven and earth do not give the feeling of change. They give the feeling of two separate entities rather than the play between them. But the hexagrams or trigrams always refer to the change between the two, and life is within that change.

When heaven and earth are duplicated this gives the four seasons, and the four seasons are also *yin yang* but seen as four. Putting the two and the four together you have the six which are called the six junctions, and a junction is not the physical entering of this or that, but the idea of blowing and diffusing one towards the other. This idea is given in Zhuangzi where it is said that 'living beings are blowing one towards another'.

This idea of the six junctions is a way to sum up not only the limitations of physical space, but a way to understand the limitation through the exchanges of *qi*.

The six junctions are used as an image of the visible world which is reproduced in each of us as the bodily frame. So whether we are talking about the universe or talking about ourselves there is no difference, the laws are equally true. It is really this exchange of *qi* which is seen by the author, because *qian* and *kun*, east and west, south and north are not so much directions but the ways and the places in which *qi* is exchanged.

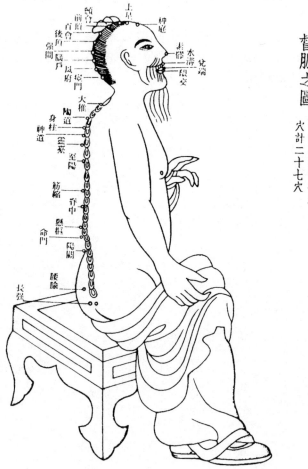

Du mai from the Neiwaigong tushuo

DU MAI 督脈

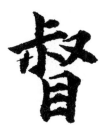

Elisabeth Rochat: In Wieger's Chinese Characters (lesson 124) the upper part of the character *du* (叔) is given as collecting beans, but this meaning was quite obsolete even in classical times. The character developed the meaning of uncle or more precisely, the father's younger brother, or the husband's younger brother. The lower part (目) represents an eye.

The meaning of the complete character is governor, but what kind of governor? It is a man, for instance a younger brother, who has the responsibility to 'look out' for his elder brother. Thinking in terms of an empire or a kingdom, it would be something like a viceroy. In India at the time of the Raj, the viceroy was generally a man connected to the royal family. In China there would have been a viceroy for example in Canton, and generally he would be a member of the emperor's family because that would be more secure.

This kind of governor is in charge, because he is close to the supreme general power, he is like a delegate. So *du* has all these associated meanings – to control, to watch over, to rule, to stimulate and also to correct. He is the commander-in-chief of the armed forces, a viceroy, or a man in charge of overseeing in a particular area.

The phonetic (叔), which is the upper part, can be put together with other radicals and get some interesting meanings. For example, with the radical for water (淑) it means good pure water, or something very clear and pure; if used to describe a person, it is someone who is full of virtue, excellent, fine, good and even skilful. With the radical for woman (婌) it is a special title for the governess of the women in the royal palace, not only the maids, but the ladies-in-waiting and the concubines. She has authority over all the women. Adding the cloth radical (裻) gives the idea of a seam, especially the seam in the middle of the back of a garment. Even in quite ancient times this seam was the symbol of the middle way and the right way to follow. This appears in Zhuangzi chapter 3, The Secret of Caring for Life, when he is advising to follow the middle way:

> 'Your life has a limit but knowledge has none. If you use what is limited to pursue what has no limit, you will be in danger. If you understand this and still strive for knowledge, you will be in danger for certain! If you do good, stay away from fame. If you do evil, stay away from punishments. Follow the middle (*du* 督); go by what is constant, and you can stay in one piece, keep yourself alive, look after your parents, and live out your years.'
>
> [based on Burton Watson's translation]

To 'follow the middle' is follow the *du* (督) which is like a rule, and rule in Zhuangzi may also be *jing* (經), the term we use for meridian.

So even in the first and second centuries BC, this character *du* already had the meaning of something very strong, something very constant, able to give a guideline for life. This is important when we compare it to the meaning of *ren* (任). If we use the same radicals with the phonetic *ren*, of *ren mai*, it gives quite a different meaning to each character.

The Chinese classical texts also explain this character *du* with another of the same sound, an homophone; and if there is an analogy of a sound, there is often an analogy of meaning. This other *du* (都) is a great town, a capital city, an administrative centre, and it is from this centre that the kingdom is able to flourish, become rich and prosperous. The explanation is that a capital city or an administrative centre is like the main rope of a net which holds all the other smaller strings in place. This is the comparison with the *du mai*.

Another character used to express the essential quality of *du mai* is *gang* (綱), the same character which is used in the term *ba gang* (八 綱), the eight principles, where the image is also of this great rope of a net. But the abstract meaning is more the principle of something. You can see that through this use of the character, *du mai* is like the director and the place from where all different forms of expression can be ruled. For all the *yang* functions within the body, it is the administrative centre, the principle, the main rope for all the *yang mai*; not only the *yang* meridians, but all the circulation which is an expression of the *yang* power. It is where all the *yang qi* is mastered. Another name for *du mai* is the sea of the *yang mai*. Another is to be a supervisor, to gather into a unity – to be like a leader, to preside over something, as a general supervisor of all the *yang* functions of the body.

Claude Larre: If we were discussing the heart, our vocabulary would be different, it would be higher, but we are talking of *qi* and the network of vital circulation. We are not concerned here with the higher level of authority which is presided over by the heart. That is why there is this aspect of being second best, not to put this governor in a place that is too high, but to keep him in his proper place. The prime minister is not the king. The prime minister is only the prime minister. We have to be careful with all these ranks. This man is overseeing everything, but he is looking on behalf of someone else. He is the viceroy, the delegate and only that.

THE PATHWAY OF DU MAI

Elisabeth Rochat: In looking at the pathway of *du mai* we will try to see the significance of its function and role. The simplest description is in Nanjing difficulty 28:

> '*Du mai* rises from the *yu* (俞) of the lower ridge pole (*xia ji* 下 極); it doubles the spinal column on the inside; it rises to *feng fu* (風 府 Du 16) and penetrates the brain with

which it takes a belonging relationship.'

So what is the meaning of this character *yu* (俞)? Generally it is the designation of an acupuncture point; a place where something can pass from the exterior, for example the stimulation from an acupuncture needle, to the inner function of the body, or from the inner viscera towards the surface. The etymology of the character suggests a boat floating and following the current of a river. Point is not a very good translation – it is more the place where something is conveyed.

Du mai begins at Du 1, *chang qiang* (長 強), though in some sources it is said to begin at Ren 1, *hui yin* (會 陰). But what is this lower ridge pole? If we look at the beginning of *ren mai* it is clear that this tern is used to give a symmetrical presentation to *du mai* and *ren mai*. The author of the Nanjing wanted to emphasize this ridge pole (*ji* 極) as the starting point of *du mai* and *ren mai*, in order to show how these two meridians provide the first unity of the body before it begins to take shape. The expression *tai ji* (太 極), supreme ridge pole, had a very significant meaning at the time of the writing of the Nanjing; it was seen as the supreme point of attachment for everything that exists.

Claude Larre: This reflects back to the *liu he* (六 合), the six junctions. We can choose to take the view of the individual within the universe, or the universe within the individual. The individual being is in the centre of everything, as that is a fact of our consciousness, but the limitation of our individual selves within the universe is not known. When we speak of the supreme this or the supreme that, it means both the highest level of the universe and the beginning of our own life. And it is impossible to make a localization of the point where life is given or where life ceases to act within us. We must make a distinction between life which is visible, and life which is functioning but invisible.

Elisabeth Rochat: The *tai ji*, the supreme ridge pole of the universe, exists before the first division into *yin* and *yang*. These are the broken and unbroken lines of the Yijing. Then come the four images, the eight trigrams and the 64 hexagrams. This vision is a reflection of the thought of the Han dynasty, which is the period of the Nanjing. The *ji* (極 ridge pole) is seen as the beginning of the *du mai* and the *ren mai*, and this is in order to convey the idea of the first division into *yin* and *yang* from the primitive unity, where there is no shape and no form. The character *xia* (下 lower), is used here because it is only from the depths of the earth that something can rise up and move towards heaven. This is a *yang* movement of rising up and extending.

Some commentators say that the first point of *du mai* is *hui yin* (會 陰), Ren 1. The character *hui* (會) suggests a great gathering of *yin*, a great meeting in the *yin* area of the body, which sometimes means the sexual organs, sometimes just the lower part of the abdomen. If we take this meaning we can understand *hui yin* as the meeting of all the mysterious power of life coming from the depths of the belly. *Hui yin* as well as *chang qiang* (長 強 Du 1) are projections of the mystery of life in the lower abdomen towards the exterior.

Claude Larre: We must remember that with the eight extraordinary meridians we are dealing with this primitive embryonic aspect of life. If we were talking about the kidneys it would be different, and of course the starting point of the meridian would be on the foot. But the *ren* and *du mai* are concerned with a development before that of the four limbs, so the starting point must be at the base of the trunk. And at this stage we cannot separate the *ren mai* and the *du mai* as they are still interconnected.

Elisabeth Rochat: We will see later that different commentators give other possible starting points inside the body, but the common starting point for both *ren* and *du mai* is often given as *hui yin* (Ren 1), and the mysterious origin of *ren mai, du mai* and *chong mai* is within the body in this kind of vital envelope in the lower abdomen.

'...It doubles the spinal column on the inside. It rises to *feng fu* (風 府 Du 16).'

This is not the description of a superficial pathway, but a deep one. *Du mai* is on the back, and if it is said to be doubling the spinal column, this suggests that it gives strength to the back bone, which is the core of the trunk of the body. It rises to *feng fu* (風 府 Du 16, Storehouse of the Wind), but why do they choose this point? *Feng fu* is at the end of the spinal column, between the spinal column, the skull and the brain. Wind (*feng* 風) is often used to describe the breath of life, or the *qi*. Long before it was used in relation to perverse energy, wind described the impetuosity of life, or the *yang* movement of life and its ability to move quickly and over a distance – it is to put something in motion. This is probably why this point is chosen here.

Du mai has an ascending movement, and the strength of this movement is visible in the hardness of the bones. Through *feng fu* all these strong influences penetrate the brain, bringing *yang* and spiritual stimulation. The brain is a mass of *yin* and it needs the inspiration of the *yang* and the light of the spirits to be energized. It needs clarity for the upper orifices to function, and through the upper orifices the ability to perceive, know and adapt to the exterior world.

The special relationship between *du mai* and the brain is a *shu* (屬), belonging, relationship: this means to be, by one's nature, under the authority of something. They depend one upon the other, they belong together, and this relationship is the same as that of each of the twelve meridians with its own organ, the lung meridian with the lungs and so on. We will see later that the *du mai* has other relationships with other functions within the body, but in its ascending movement it has this belonging relationship with the *yin* of the brain. It rises from the *yin* in the lower part of the trunk and ends in the *yin* in the upper part. And this upper *yin*, the brain, is the appropriate receptacle for the finest *yang* influences coming from this other original mixing in the depths.

SUWEN CHAPTER 60

'...*Du mai* arises in the lower abdomen and descends directly in the middle of the bone (symphysis pubis). In women it penetrates to connect with the extremity of the urinary meatus. Its *luo* (絡) passes through the vase of *yin* (sexual organs) and makes a junction (*he* 合) between the two lower orifices at the perineum. It follows the curve of the perineum behind and through a detachment (*bie* 別) follows the curve of the buttocks; it reaches the *shao yin* (kidney meridian) as well as the central *luo* of the great *yang* (bladder meridian). It makes a junction with the *shao yin*, and rises on the upper internal face of the thigh; it passes through the spinal column and takes a relation of dependence (*shu* 屬) with the kidneys.

'It arises with the *tai yang* in the internal corner of the eye, rises to the forehead and makes a crossing (*jiao* 交) above the top of the head (*dian* 巔); it penetrates and takes a connecting (*luo* 絡) relationship with the brain; its detachment (*bie* 別) descends to the nape of the neck. It passes through the internal part of the scapula, flanks the spinal column and reaches the middle of the loins; it penetrates and runs along the vertebral column and takes a connecting (*luo* 絡) relationship with the kidneys. In *men* it runs along the penis and descends to the perineum; then it is the same as for women.

'The pathway that rises directly from the lower abdomen runs through the middle of the navel, rises to go through the heart and penetrates the throat; rises to the chin, encircles the lips and rises to connect under both eyes, right in the middle.'

Elisabeth Rochat: This is obviously not the usual pathway rising from Du 1 to the summit of the head, and then descending to the inner lips at Du 28. We will see, especially in the Suwen, that this point Du 28 may be seen as a point of *ren mai*. The present assignation of points to particular meridians is quite recent.

This text describes three trajectories of *du mai*, one in the lower part of the trunk, beginning in the lower abdomen, and commentators in later texts identified this as the 'intimate envelope', *bao* (胞). The meaning of this character *bao* (胞) is of a matrix, a very precious wrapping of something. For women it is the special envelope for new life which we call the uterus and which is one of the six extraordinary *fu*. But men and women both have this *bao*, so it is not only the uterus, but also the way in which individual vitality is guarded and held at the origin within lower abdomen. This *bao* has a very strong link with the kidneys, in this case with the kidneys as the keeper of original *yin* and *yang*, authentic fire and water and so on. *Bao* both protects the individual life and the mysterious point from which the division and differentiation of *qi* bursts out. The term *bao zhong* (胞 中) is often used to suggest the centre where life is protected.

Some texts describe the origin of *du mai*, *ren mai* and *chong mai* as this well protected centre, or as in the lower abdomen, or the area of the kidneys, and it is all much the same idea, because it is not possible to give a precise location for *bao* when it is just this concept of the mysterious beginning of life, and the way it is preserved.

From this joint beginning, the *du mai* descends directly in the middle of the bone, *heng gu,* meaning horizontal bone (as in the name of the point Kidney 11), or the pubic symphysis. The backbone is the best example of verticality in the body, of the ascending *yang* power, with *du mai* and the *tai yang* bladder meridian. This backbone is like a vertical column, but in the front it is the opposite, the horizontal bone, *heng gu*, the symphysis pubis, and also the hyoid. In the vision of the body, both real and symbolic, there is always an opposition between the back and the front, between *du mai* and *ren mai*, between the *yang* and the *yin*, and between the verticality of the *qi* and the *yang* and the horizontality of the earth and the *yin*. So at the front of the body there is this supporting bone, and at this level both *ren mai* and *du mai*, make a network of communication in the perineum and have a relationship with the two lower orifices.

In this area there is a close relationship with the kidney meridian, and also a strong influence of *du mai* on the sexual organs, because the sexual organs are not only governed by *yin*, but need the *yang* to move the *yin*. We know that problems in the lower abdomen are not only because of *yin* deficiency, emptiness of blood for example, but also because of an emptiness of *qi*. There are many examples of that relating to the pathology of *du mai* later in this chapter.

'...It follows the curve of the perineum behind and through a detachment (*bie* 別) follows the curve of the buttocks;

it reaches the *shao yin* (kidney meridian) as well as the central *luo* of the great *yang* (bladder meridian).'

'The central *luo* of the great *yang*' is just another way to say the bladder meridian. This is the area of Bladder 35, *hui yang* (會 陽), which is a meeting of the *yang*, a kind of exit from the *yin* to the *yang*, at the beginning of the spinal column. Here something is completed, something from the lower abdomen moving in a kind of loop, passing through the genitals and the lower part of the spinal column.

'...It makes a junction with the *shao yin*, and rises on the upper internal face of the thigh; it passes through the spinal column and takes a relation of dependence with the kidneys.'

This is the same as the description of the bladder meridian given in Lingshu chapter 10. In the lower part, *du mai* is central, then as it follows the curve of the buttock it becomes bilateral – perhaps having a special relationship with the kidney meridian. It is important that we think of this meridian as affecting the whole area rather than as a thread or a single line. The single central line is more like a symbol of the effectiveness of *du mai*.

'...It arises with the *tai yang* in the internal corner of the eye, it rises to the forehead and makes a crossing (*jiao* 交) above the head; it penetrates taking a *luo* relation with the brain; returning, it detaches (*bie* 別) and descends to the nape of the neck. It passes through the internal part of the scapula, flanks the spinal column and reaches the middle of the loins; it penetrates and runs along the vertebral column and takes a connecting (*luo* 絡) relationship with the kidneys. In men it runs along the penis and descends to the perineum; then it is the same as for women.'

It has a *luo* connection with the brain which is the same relationship as each meridian has with its associated viscera, for example, the spleen meridian with the stomach, the lung meridian with the large intestine. It also has a *luo* relationship with the kidneys. As it ascends it has a *shu* belonging relationship, and as it descends it has a *luo* relationship. Finally there is a third trajectory in the middle of the belly. Coming from the lower abdomen through the navel, through the heart and rising up to the area under the centre of the eye, which is the traditional ending for *ren mai*.

'...The pathway that rises directly from the lower abdomen runs through the middle of the navel, rises to go through the heart and penetrates the throat; it rises to the chin, encircles the lips and rises to connect under the eyes, right in the middle.'

All the great *yang* centres of movement, the original *qi* and the original fire, are represented in the first trajectory within the lower abdomen. The kidneys provide another expression of the origin; original *yang* and original *yin*. In the brain the finest and most subtle *yang qi* accumulates. The clear *yang* rises up to allow the superior function of the brain and the upper orifices, facilitating communication with heaven and the exterior in the most subtle way through the orifices –

the eyes, the ears and the nose. There are strong references to the communication between the brain and the eyes, and between the brain and the nose in the text of the Suwen, and many commentators emphasize the role of *du mai* in respiration, and the descending movement from the nose down to the kidneys. This is perhaps the foundation of the function of the kidneys to attract the *qi* of the respiration down to the base of the trunk. This is not only the embryonic respiration mentioned in daoist alchemical texts, but also the foundation of one of the functions of the *zang* and *fu*.

The eyes are very important because they represent the *yang* in the upper orifices, they are like the sun in the human body. The eyes open during the day and close during the night, giving rhythm to the appearance and disappearance of the light, the sun and the *yang*. This is why in the adult the rhythm of the *wei qi*, the defensive *qi*, is mastered from the eyes, and the *qiao mai*, which are linked with *du mai* and *ren mai*, are in charge of these regulations at another stage of development.

The eyes are also the place of *zong mai* (宗 脈), the ancestral circulation – ancestral with the meaning of gathering together in order to have a place for a unified mastery or ruling. The same character is used for *zong qi* (宗 氣), the ancestral *qi*, and it suggests the ability to hold firmly and master a function of the body. Here at the eyes there is a mastery of the network of animation, because so many meridians and *luo* meet at the eyes, begin in the area around the eyes, or even pass through the eyes, like the liver meridian. *Du mai* provides the first organization for this.

There is also a relationship between *du mai* and the navel, which expresses a relationship with the mother, a relationship which is not only physical, but psychic and perhaps spiritual at the deepest level. The name of the point of *ren mai* at the navel is *shen que* (神 闕 Spirit Watchtower, Ren mai 8). *Que* suggests a breach or an opening of the wall around a city which allows movement in and out. Some commentators studying this point say that the name comes from the fact that the child first receives its spirits from the mother through the umbilical cord; it is a passage for the spirits. The navel is important not only for the *yin* part of the body, but also for the penetration of the spirits and the *qi*. That is the reason that *du mai* is represented in this area.

After that, the heart is also mentioned in this description of the pathway of *du mai*. The heart is seen as the great *yang*, in charge of all circulation and networks of animation, the emperor fire and the ministerial fire. It is an expression of the *yang* power of the spirit inside the body, which manifests itself through the power of circulation and animation. Of course the *ren mai* also has a very strong relationship with the heart because the heart is master of the blood. The pathway then reaches the throat, which is a passage for the breath. The *du mai* rises to the chin and finally collects under the two eyes, in the centre below each eye.

So what is the meaning of this strange description? *Du mai* is that which is able to gather, to unify and to master the *yang qi* of the whole body and at the same time ensure the communication and relationships from the administrative centre of the *yang qi* in the body of the adult. This also implies the connection of the *yang* power of the *qi* in the body and the origin of the *yang* power in the kidneys, *ming men* and lower abdomen. Because it is present in all these different areas of the body, *du mai* is able to control, harmonize and regulate, and at the same time give life and stimulate the *qi* and the *yang* of the whole body.

Some commentators suggest that the two different relationships with the kidneys, one with the ascending pathway and the other with the descending pathway, draw attention to a double relationship with the *yin* and *yang* of the two kidneys, the left and the right, or the kidneys and *ming men*. These ideas are expressed in the Nanjing, particularly in difficulties 36 and 39. In this context, commentators say that the first pathway, the rising trajectory, begins in the *yin* in the depths of the lower abdomen, the genitals, the mysterious hidden part of the vitality, rises through the spinal column and backbone and has a *shu* relationship with the kidneys.

Certain commentators point out that this is the right kidney which corresponds to *ming men*, and that it is a movement from the *yin* towards a relationship with the *yang*. Conversely, the descending pathway begins in the *yang* part of the body and at the exterior, and is seen as the manifestation of the *yang* vitality descending to take a *luo* relationship with the left kidney which is the *yin* kidney, the water. So this is coming from the *yang* and descending to have a relationship with the *yin*.

This implies that *du mai* is related to the *yang* of the kidneys and has a kind of associate relationship with the *yin*, but it is most important to see that *du mai* has an influence in each of the areas of the body where the *yang* power is active and has an area of command. The *yang qi* of the human body, the defensive *qi*, rises from the lower abdomen and has a relationship with the eyes. It is this inspiration and clarification by the *yang* in the lower abdomen which forms the *wei qi*. And it is the function of the *yang qi* in the body that gives a relationship between *wei qi* and *du mai*.

The *du mai*, through this mastery of the *yang*, is also like a supervisor of all the *yang* vitality in each of the *zang fu* – through the circulation of the twelve meridians, all the organization of the *zang* and *fu* and the relationships between them. But even though the *du mai* is the master of *yang* it also has very strong relationships with the *yin*, with the front of the body, and with the kidneys, because in the building of the human body there must always be a conjunction of *yin* and *yang*. Nothing on earth is pure *yang* or pure *yin*, and even *du mai*, which in a way is the purest expression of *yang* in the body, has this constant interrelationship with the *yin*. So *du mai* is the first of the extraordinary meridians, logically speaking, because its influence is seen everywhere.

Question: Could you relate the *du mai* to the first division of the cell after conception? There is some idea that the place in the body where that begins is the equivalent of *ming men*. Is there anything suggesting this in the texts?

Elisabeth Rochat: Not at the level of the cell, no. It is the beginning of differentiation, yes, but that is not developed and discussed in the Chinese medical texts. But I think it is possible to interpret that.

Claude Larre: You may build images in your own mind which relate to your own understanding, but we cannot expect the Chinese to come to such a speculation, especially at the level of the cell. They were more concerned with the general direction of life than in making an investigation into how one cell may be dividing at the very beginning. And if we make this comparison, it may help our own understanding, but it certainly has no grounding in the Chinese text. The Chinese text is concerned with the opposition – that one is for overseeing, the other is for sustaining, the one for injecting the life power, the other to make sure that it is contained somewhere. And that is the only way that we can answer the question. Other additional remarks can only be in the mind of the commentator.

Elisabeth Rochat: These eight meridians are more primitive and original than the twelve, and within the eight meridians those which are most extraordinary and unique are the *du mai, ren mai, chong mai* and *dai mai*. The first four extraordinary meridians do not exactly have a pathway, but they express the first organization of *yin* and *yang* in the body; in the case of *du mai*, the *yang* power and its distribution. This is the reason why the *du mai* is the master of the *yang*, of all the *yang* meridians and all the *yang* circulation. Not only that, but it also masters all the *yang* command points. It is because of this that it is original, because it is the first organizer, able to take all the areas of organization of the *yang* together. After that it is more differentiated, more particular.

Question: In some respects this frontal pathway of *du mai* seems to have hijacked the pathway of *ren mai*, can you comment on that?

Elisabeth Rochat: We will see that *ren mai* also has a trajectory in the back; *chong mai* too. And they have the same starting point. *Du mai* expresses the *yang* power enveloping and animating the whole body except for the four limbs. *Ren mai* is in the front but also goes towards the back, as does the *chong mai*. The difference is not so much in the trajectory or pathway but in the fact that the *du mai* is more in charge of the *yang* aspect, movement and *qi*, and *ren mai* is in charge of the *yin* aspect, blood and fluids, and to support and maintain. For example, the spirits need both essences and *qi*, the heart needs blood as well *qi*, essences as well as movement. The kidneys also have these two aspects of *yin* and *yang*, water and fire, and I think that it is in the establishment of these main areas of *yang* influence and areas of *yin* influence that we see the importance of *ren* and *du mai*.

There is never absolute *yang* and absolute *yin*, and the *yin* and the *yang*, the *du mai* and the *ren mai*, have very strong connections and relationships. They are undifferentiated at the level of the origin, like chaos, and then it is a matter of function as to which areas fall under the influence of *ren mai* or *du mai*. When we speak of blood, we are in the area of influence of *ren mai* and *chong mai*, but if we are talking of the dynamism of *qi*, and the ability to move and circulate the blood effectively then we are more concerned with *du mai*. *Ren mai* and *chong mai* give the richness of the essences to the quality of the blood and define the areas where they go. The force of the circulation is given by the *yang*. The *tai ji* diagram shows the first stage of the *yin* within the *yang*, the *yang* within the *yin*, and that is the same in the human body with the interpenetration and doubling of *du mai* and *ren mai*.

In Suwen chapter 60, the movement of the *du mai* emerges from the original breath and then rises – repeating in part the description of the pathway of the bladder meridian, *tai yang* of the foot. This is in order to show the other *yang* function in the body, which is not only an ascending movement but also the power to descend with a kind of pressure – because *qi* and movement are present throughout the body, not only for ascending but also for descending. All these movements are controlled by the *yang*. So this part of the description just repeats the pathway of the bladder meridian, and in a way the bladder meridian, together with the *du mai*, express this power of the vertical axis on the back. And of course all the *shu* points of the viscera are on the bladder meridian just as there are many *mu* points on the *ren mai* at the front.

As far as the spine is concerned, what meridians have a relationship with the spinal column? The bladder and the kidneys of course, but also the three tendon-muscular meridians of the stomach, spleen and large intestine. I am not suggesting any theories about that, just giving you the information, but there does seem to be some kind of relationship with the power of spleen and stomach and post-heaven in their renewal of *qi* in the organism. In the same way the *ren mai* has a relationship with the spleen and stomach for the renewal of essences and blood. The *chong mai* also has a very strong relationship with the stomach and the kidneys, but from a different point of view, because the relationship of *du mai* with all these parts is in order to manifest the presence of the *yang* power and to master it. The *ren mai* does the same for the *yin*. *Chong mai* manifests the unity of *yin* and *yang*.

Let us look at a text from the Yuan dynasty (13th-14th C):

> '*Du* and *ren mai* have one unique string, one is in the front of the body the other in the back of the body, and there is the possibility of division and junction. You can divide them or you can join them. When one divides them, after a while one sees that *yin* and *yang* never leave each other. When one joins them, then after a while one sees that it is like chaos without distinction like the primitive and original mixing of everything.'

We can see *ren mai* and *du mai* in differentiation or in unity. But if we are concerned with differentiation, we have to return to the unity; in unity we remain in the chaotic vision of origin, or come back to differentiation. In making differentiation, *yin* is on the front and the *yang* on the back, but this is always coming from the more chaotic state of unity. *Ren* and *du mai* are produced from original *qi* (*yuan qi* 元氣) and for this reason we can understand the important role of *du mai* and *ren mai* in all forms of daoist meditation. This is the perfect way to remain in good health – to understand both the unity and the differentiation; to be able to circulate the blood and *qi* well, while not leaving the unity of your own body, and by this kind of exercise to understand the body as part of the cosmos. But this is for those in good health!

Question: Could you clarify the direction of energy flow in the *du mai*?

Elisabeth Rochat: According to the Neijing and a lot of other texts, the most usual way to describe the *du mai* is as an ascending movement from the perineum to the top of the head and then to the eyes and mouth. Because this is a symbolic representation of the *yang* power, giving vertical strength to the body and acting as the axis of the *yang* exchange.

But I think that the direction, the ascending or descending movement described here is symbolic of the double function of both ascending and descending. This means that there is not only an ascending movement in the back and an descending movement in the front, but more that because the *yin* energy must rise up there must be an ascending movement at the front, and to emphasize the fact that the *yang* also has to descend, the movement of *du mai* also descends at the back.

I do not know if it is more strange to think of *ren mai* and *du mai* with this kind of doubling, or to imagine a body, with a common origin, suddenly making a complete division in the area of the perineum into *yin* and *yang*. Which is the most strange? Both are true in their own way. But you must understand that this is not a separation, just an expression of the duality of the way in which *du mai* and *ren mai* control *yin* and *yang*, blood and *qi*, fire and water within this first division of vitality. It is the same as the kidneys, they are double or they are one. It depends.

PATHOLOGY OF DU MAI

Suwen chapter 60 presents several pathologies of *du mai*. One is given just before the presentation of the trajectory, the other just after.

> 'When *du mai* gives rise to illness, the spinal column stiffens and is as if broken, (against the flow).'

This is very similar to the description given in Nanjing difficulty 29:

> 'When *du mai* gives rise to illnesses, the spinal column stiffens and there is withdrawal, *jue* (厥).'

Jue (厥) is a kind of weakness from withdrawal. There is not enough correct *qi* to rule the whole body and for this reason a distortion, a lack of transformation or aggressive action from the exterior is able to penetrate and gain ground – either gradually, or suddenly – it depends on the situation. This is the meaning of the character *jue*. This kind of illness concerns the pathway of *du mai* on the back of the body, but also the way in which *du mai* is able to ensure the correct circulation and good balance in the strength of the *yang qi*. For example, 'the spinal column stiffens, and is as if broken' describes an illness that is caused by a lack of regulation of the *yang qi* in the back, and there are two types. One is a perverse fullness which creates a kind of over-tension in the bones and particularly in the muscular attachments to the spine. This is because the pressure of the perverse *qi* creates a kind of swelling, which then creates pressure causing stiffness and pain as if the back is broken.

But it is possible to have the same symptoms due to an emptiness of *yang qi*. If the *yang qi* is empty the back is very vulnerable, especially to all kinds of attack from wind and cold. In this case, if the *yang qi* is weakened and empty it is unable to warm the spinal column and the bones and marrow inside. There is a lack of defensive *qi* and penetration by perverse energies of cold or wind could also create stiffness. Of course we must make the distinction whether the cause of the pain is fullness or emptiness. It may be due to a general emptiness of *yang* in the body or due to blockage, obstruction and congestion.

Later in Suwen 60 it says:

> 'When illnesses are produced from the lower abdomen (in connection with the *du mai*) it rises to rush (*chong* 衝) at the heart and cause pain there; one cannot go either in front or behind (neither urine or stool). This is *shan* (疝) syndrome with an impetuous current (*chong shan* 衝 疝). In women there is sterility, dysuria, haemorrhoids, urinary incontinence, dry throat.

'When *du mai* produces its illnesses, one treats *du mai*;
one treats above the bone, when it is serious one treats at
the power of the constitution, which is under the navel.'

'Above the bone' refers to Ren 2 (*qu gu* 曲 骨) and the other
indication below the navel is for Ren 7 (*yin qiao* 陰 交), which
according to the Nanjing is the special command point of the
lower heater.

This pathology is not only linked with *du mai*, but with the
joint pathways of *ren mai*, *du mai* and *chong mai*, which
control the lower abdomen and ensure circulation and the
correct balance between the ascending and descending
movement of blood and *qi* and fluids. It is important for
blood and fluids to circulate well in order to ensure the
correct functioning of the lower orifices, as well as all the
elements of vitality in the depths of the abdomen, especially
for reproduction. *Du mai* governs the ability to raise the
vitality from the lower part of the body up to the upper
abdomen and the upper part of the thorax, to the heart and
the throat, and so on.

All this pathology is a kind of counter-current, meaning
that the *qi*, the *yang*, is too strong, and unable to remain in
correct balance with the *yin* in the lower abdomen; the rising
up movement is too strong. This is the reason for this kind
of rush at the heart, causing cardialgia or pains in the heart.
We must remember from the earlier descriptions that *du mai*
and of course *ren mai* and *chong mai* too, have a relationship
with the heart and the upper heater, and if there is a counter-
current, the circulation of blood and fluids will be disturbed.

For instance, sterility for women may be because the blood, under the authority of the heart, is unable to descend and enrich the inner abdomen, where fertility in women resides. So this kind of disturbance can cause sterility in women.

The lower orifices, which are under the authority of *du mai* and *ren mai*, may also lack the power necessary to contain and to hold, because the *yang* is rising too strongly. This would cause urinary incontinence and haemorrhoids due to stagnation and bad circulation. The throat, where *du mai*, *ren mai* and *chong mai* pass through, would be dry, because fluids are not carried up to the throat, and by the same movement of the *yang*, they may be dried up. The movement and agitation of the *yang* which harms the heart, can also dry up the fluids in the brain and upper orifices. We can see this in the name and function of the points on the *ren mai*, for example Ren 22 (*tian tu* 天 突) and Ren 23 (*lian quan* 廉 泉) are very strong points for the circulation of fluids in the upper parts of the body.

So we can see that this is not exactly a pathology of *du mai* or a pathology of *ren mai*, it is a pathology of the correct balance between them – between blood and *qi* and the circulation of blood and *qi* in this part of the body where all the vitality is hidden, reproduction is centred, and the nutrition of the heart and all the viscera is maintained. Treatment is on the *ren mai*, with the two points which balance the lower heater, the meeting place of the *yin* and *yang* at the level of the origin.

Question: What is *shan* (疝)?

Elisabeth Rochat: It can refer to all kinds of hernia, but it is not only that. The character is made with the radical for illness and the phonetic for mountain (山). There are two meanings for this mountain, it can be a protuberance, which, like a mountain is visible externally, but it can also be a kind of accumulation of stones or of earth piled up. Many diseases of the lower heater linked to bad circulation can also be called *shan*, whether due to lack of defensive *qi*, congestion or blockage or any kind of accumulation. Hernia is just one of the interpretations. Generally there is another character before *shan* to give the precise meaning. *Chong shan* (衝 疝) is a kind of stagnation, blockage and cold in the lower abdomen caused by an aggressive rising of *qi*, also giving symptoms in the upper heater and the throat; it is a kind of separation of *yin* and *yang*, which is the main point of this pathology.

HEADACHES

There are also other classical pathologies of *du mai*, including headaches or a feeling of heaviness in the head. This may be due to an emptiness of *yang* or an emptiness of *yin* creating false strength of the *yang*. In the first instance of the emptiness and weakness of the *yang qi*, the deficiency is in the ability of the clear *yang* (*qing yang* 清 陽) to rise up through the *du mai*. This clear *yang* is pure enough to invigorate the brain and the upper orifices, which is one of the main functions of *du mai* – to enable the clear *yang qi* to reach its goal in the upper part of the body. If the *du mai* is too weak to do that, if the *yang qi* is too weak, the *qi* will not be clear enough and does not have enough strength to reach the brain and animate this mass of *yin* in the head. This is why there is the feeling of heaviness in the head.

If, on the contrary, the *yang* is too strong, it may cause imbalance between the *yin* and the *yang*, and there will be an upward counter-current. In this case the excess *yang* will cause agitation and movement. Because it is not stabilized by the *yin*, the *yang* causes problems in the upper part of the body, not exactly a heavy head, but a headache with agitation, and pain. Both of these kinds of headaches may be connected with *du mai*.

MANIA AND DEMENTIA

According to many texts, *du mai* pathology includes dementia and mania, *dian kuang* 癲 狂. In this context *dian* is seen as a *yin* madness, *kuang* a *yang* madness. The lack or weakness of *yang* and *qi* causes an abundance of *yin* and phlegm; there is no inflammation, just congestion due to dampness and untransformed fluids, occupying the interior of the trunk. When this congestion reaches the level of the upper heater, there is an insufficiency in the spirits and consciousness due to the lack of *yang qi* and insufficient support of the *du mai* to the heart: they are not animated by the *yang*. At the same time there is blockage and heaviness due to untransformed fluids. This is the cause of dementia (*dian* 癲) and the main symptoms are that behaviour and thinking are not clear but disordered and without consistency. The person may laugh and cry alternatively.

Mania, *kuang* 狂, is quite the contrary. It is the super-abundance of perverse *yang*, fire and heat. In this case the phlegm is accompanied by inflammation, it is very dense and thick, and congests the orifices of the heart. The agitation of the heart and in the upper heater generally creates a disturbance in the expression of the spirits; there is agitation and anger, which is often compared to a bolting horse.

Question: Can this be related to epilepsy?

Elisabeth Rochat: Epilepsy can be a result of this same process, and some texts say that this pathology of *du mai* applies to adults, whereas for children there may be convulsions or epilepsy. The reason for this is that the function of *du mai* is to regulate the *yang* and the *qi*. Here we can see both sides of the disturbance of that regulation – one too weak, one too strong. But the *du mai* is not only for the *yang* and the *qi*, it also maintains the effectiveness of the spirits, as we can see in the names of the points on the *du mai* at the level of the heart such as *shen dao* (神 道), Du 11, The Way of the Spirits.

The spirits must be present in the upper orifices and the brain, and *du mai* plays its part in the expression of the spirits by regulating the *yang* in the body. This pathology is given for adults, because the most serious injury is an injury to the expression of the spirits. In a child the symptoms may be more physical and manifest as convulsions and epilepsy.

There are many kinds of convulsions mentioned in the classical texts, but when the pulse is very weak and empty the treatment may be easier than when there is a large, swollen pulse indicating the presence of perverse energy. In this case it is a sign that the perverse wind is very strong and treatment can be difficult.

With convulsions and epilepsy, there may be other symptoms such as episthotonos, which is an excess of tension and counter-current. Du 20 (*bai hui* 百 會) is one of the points used in this case because of its relationship with the brain. Nanjing 28 mentions penetration from *feng fu* (風 府), Du 16, into the brain, and also through the pathway of the bladder meridian at Bladder 7 (*tong tian* 通 天). Deficiency of *du mai* can lead to lack of defence and a perversion of wind in the head. *Nao feng* (腦 風), 'wind in the brain', is a name for headaches or vertigo and sometimes dementia. *Bai hui* can be used in all these cases of tension, episthotonos and stiffness of the muscular attachments along the spine, as it is also the meeting point between the *du mai* and the liver meridian which is of course the master of the muscles.

Question: When would you decide to use the extraordinary meridians in treatment rather than the twelve ordinary meridians?

Elisabeth Rochat: If the *qi* and the *yang* are lacking in power, this may be very similar to the symptoms of a decrease in the fire of *ming men* (命 門) and also of the *qi* and *yang* of post-heaven. These are very general symptoms, for example a kind of withdrawal and lack of defensive *qi* coming from the origin. In the case of fullness it is like an overflow, with congestion and blockage of this *yang* pressure. It is not a question of one specific aspect, or one *zang* that is concerned, but rather an aspect of the general movement which is disturbed, either the ascending or descending movement. In the case of *du mai* there may be all kinds of disturbance of the general mastering of the *yang*. But of course there are also a lot of very specific clinical uses of the eight extraordinary meridians which can be seen as a kind of general framework for the whole body and the whole pathology. It is always a question of technical application, and not a question of being true or false. Some schools may say that the eight extraordinary meridians are for inner meditation and the twelve are for treatment. In China there are many different approaches.

POINT NAMES OF DU MAI

Elisabeth Rochat: Let us consider the movement and function of *du mai* through the names of the points. This is not intended as a complete study of the point names of the *du mai*, I have just chosen for each point the interpretation which helps us to understand this great axis of *du mai*.

Du 1 *chang qiang* 長 強

This character *qiang* (強) only occurs in one other point name, that of Du 18 (*qiang jian* 強 間). The meaning of *qiang*

(強) is strong and powerful. The meaning of *chang* (長) is of a leader or chief, and it also means long, with a great duration in space or time. *Qiang* (強) is the image of a very solid and strong bow, and it means power and vigour, and also strain and effort. In Suwen chapter 8, the charge of the kidneys is to arouse power. And the expression 'to arouse power' uses the same character *qiang, zuo qiang* (作 強). This refers to the ability of the kidneys to provide a firm basis. If a bow is very firm and strong, it has the power to shoot an arrow a long way. But it is not the shooting of the arrow which is indicated here, it is the ability to hold this dynamic tension which is within the function of the kidneys. And it is this force which is referred to in the first point of *du mai*.

If the *du mai* leads the *yang* power of the body, then as a leader it is able to create and sustain tension at the base of the trunk, in order to stimulate the rising power of the *yang*. It is because this base is strong, that the power of the clear *yang* is able to reach the upper extremity of the body. But it must also have all the control of an archer drawing a bow. Of course archery was a great art in ancient China. You have to be very strong, and also have the ability to control this strength.

This is a very good image for the first point of the *du mai*. It suggests the strength needed to sustain the uprightness of the backbone and the ability to circulate the *qi* to all the meridians. It is the place where the strength of the *du mai* is able to reside, to rest, and it is the beginning of the rising up movement to heaven. Most of the indications of this point can be understood in this way. One of the ancient indications is long standing amenorrhoea, and needling stimulates the *yang* power and restores the proper blood circulation. All the tension and stimulation of the *yang* is located here, and when needling the point care must be taken not to cause exhaustion, which may be the case if the amenorrhoea is due to deficiency of blood. Just above this is the bladder point *hui yang* (會 陽 Bl 35) and this whole area at the base of the coccyx may be seen as a gathering of the power of the *yang*.

Du 2   *yao yu*   腰 俞

The character *yu* (俞) refers to a place from which something is sent and has an effect. *Yao* (腰) is the loins. Without the flesh radical, which denotes a part of the body, it has the meaning of essential, a key position, which is also used in military vocabulary. The loins in the body are a strategic place, not only because of the pulling in of the waist, but also because it is the place corresponding to the kidneys, the power of *ming men* and many other important points.

It is at this point that energy can be sent to provide a good basis for the area of the loins. It is a continuation of the power of the vitality of Du 1.

Du 3   *yao yang guan*   腰 陽 關

This point may be written *yao yang guan*, or simply *yang guan*. and again we have the character for the loins. This point does not appear in the old Chinese text books, but was mentioned for the first time in the Tang dynasty and became a normal point of *du mai* during the Song dynasty. This does not mean that it did not exist before, but this is the first time that it is referred to in a book. The name of the point is interesting. Again we are concerned with this power of the loins, and this time the *yang* (陽) is passing through a gateway or a pass, *guan* (關).

At Du 2 there was an injection of vitality, and here there is a kind of passage of the *yang* in order to enrich and pervade this area of the lower back. The character *guan* (關) also implies the articulations of the vertebrae. The bone articulations are seen as a passage from one vertebra to another. The loins are the main area for control of the movement of the spine, and if the lower part of the spine is strong and firm the whole spine, and all the articulations throughout the spine, can be regulated by the *yang qi*. This is also seen in the name of this point. A pass is always well controlled, it is always watched over, and on the spine this is the strategic pass before arriving at *ming men*, which is the place of the precious original *qi*. This point corresponds to the point on *ren mai, guan yuan* (關 元) which is also a pass. This may all be part of the reason why in the 10th or 11th century they decided to give this name to this point of *du mai*.

Many books say that if you moxa Du 3 the heat will radiate to the whole lower abdomen and the *zang* of the belly. This is another meaning of this *yang* passage from lower heater towards the abdomen and the *zang*. And perhaps through this point there is a general warming of the *yin* interior.

If you treat here you will invigorate the effect of this *yang* warmth inside the organism.

Du 4   *ming men*   命 門

Men (門) is a door or gate. *Ming* (命) is life destiny or mandate. This point makes the connection between *du mai* and the breath of life rooted in the depths at this level. *Ming men* is not only the name of this point but also the name of the first mysterious conjunction which gives life to a new living being. It gives not only life, but also the main principles of the individual nature and the first composition of *qi* and essences (*jing qi* 精 氣) which remains the pattern for the unfolding and renewal of each living being from birth to death. When you die, you have accomplished your mandate if you have realized all the possibilities of your own nature according to the circumstances of your life. This is the meaning of *ming*. It is the link with individual destiny and accomplishment of life, which is the accomplishment of the individual nature. That is all implied in the term *ming men*.

In the embryonic respiration of daoist meditation, *ming men* and the cinnabar fields (*dan tian* 丹 田) are very important, and this whole study of meditation and embryonic respiration involves the points and pathway of *ren mai* and *du mai*. That is quite a separate study; there is a crossover but we must be careful not to mix them up. Many points on *ren mai* and *du mai* have a strong relationship with meditation techniques and inner alchemy, but it is impossible to identify them precisely because the schools are so different in their teachings. For instance, there may be six, seven or eight points on *ren mai* and *ming men* on *du mai* which are said to relate to the lower cinnabar field. Different texts seem to suggest different points.

Du 5 *xuan shu* 懸樞

Shu (樞) is a pivot, and is the same character that is seen in the title of the Lingshu. It is a pivot and also a central axis, the hinge of a door, which allows movement. *Xuan* (懸) is to be hanging from something, to be suspended. It is used in the expression 'to be suspended above the void'. And because the heart (心) appears in the lower part of the character, it can have the meaning of anxiety, when there is the feeling of a void below the heart.

The whole spinal column can be seen as a series of suspended articulations and this name can also suggest the void between each vertebra which allows movement. If something is suspended it is necessarily above an empty space, I am not suspended if I have my feet on earth. To be suspended above the void gives the possibility of movement, which is seen in all the articulatory mechanisms, and the power of the spring. There is first the idea of a pivot, and then the idea of being suspended, and being suspended implies that you are suspended in a void. The two ideas together suggest an articulation that can function perfectly. When you begin to perform *tai ji quan* there is a subtle movement in the body to find the right axis, which is also like a pivot, and also implies a kind of suspension.

Another meaning is suggested by a special use of the character *xuan* (懸), which is found in Suwen chapter 25 for example, that the destiny (*ming* 命) of humankind is suspended from heaven. Human life on earth is like being suspended from heaven. And as this point follows *ming men*, we can infer another meaning which is a kind of ease in the movement, not only in the body and the articulations of the bones, but also in articulating the conduct of life according to one's own nature; to have the same ease, the same space and articulation for the accomplishment of the movement of one's destiny. It is very Chinese, and not only Chinese but very realistic, to have at least two levels of interpretation, because it is the same movement and the same virtue which gives the ease of movement and also gives the ease to conduct life. Because we are at the level of the foundation here. Both movement and the conduct of life are founded on the inspiration of the *yang* animation of the *du mai*. Because the *du mai* has this kind of verticality, there is a relationship with heaven and the question of how I can remain suspended from heaven in all my movements and with all my spirits.

Du 6 *ji zhong* 脊中

This is a very simple point name. *Ji* (脊) has the radical for a part of the body below (月), and a representation of the spinal column and the muscle attachments above. *Zhong* (中) is the centre. It refers to the spinal column and the idea of a centre. The most obvious interpretation is that this point is in the middle of the backbone. If we count 21 vertebrae, *ji zhong* is at the level of the 11th, between *da zhui* (大椎 Du 14) and *yao yu* (腰俞 Du 2). All the qualities of *yang qi* are needed here in order to be firm and flexible at the same time. It is also a kind of common point, being at the centre for all this flexibility and firmness of the spinal column and its muscular attachments. Remember that in Lingshu chapter 10 the bladder meridian, *tai yang* of the foot, is said to control all the diseases attacking the muscles.

Du 7 *zhong shu* 中樞

Before the 20th century many Chinese authors considered this point to be an extra point, not belonging to *du mai*. That is why some texts have only 27 points on *du mai*. The number 27 was considered more suitable for the *du mai*, as it is three times three times three. This would be a complete expression of *qi*, which is always given the number three in Chinese numerology. According to Nanjing difficulty 27 there is a discussion of the twelve main meridians and the 15 *luo* making a whole of 27 types of *qi* in the whole body. This is also mentioned in Lingshu chapter 1. The name *zhong shu* is really just a way to record the names of both the preceding points and to make a central pivot for the vitality; a pivot for movement and a centre for the movement around a common point.

Du 8 *jin suo* 筋縮

Jin (筋) is muscular strength, the kind of strength which

is able to attach the mass of flesh to the bone, especially when it is close to the bone articulation. This strength is able to mobilize the circulation within this mass of flesh and as a result give movement to the body, particularly to the limbs. Because there is no movement in the mass of flesh itself, the movement comes from the articulations and the links between the nerves and the bones and all the currents of vitality passing through the flesh. *Suo* (縮) means 'to tie together'. Sometimes it has a pathological meaning of contraction, even contraction leading to atrophy, but when it is not used pathologically, it means to hold with a link, to tie, and sometimes it means to stay in one place, or to remain in your own place, to fulfil your own function.

So we can see that this point has a double meaning. The first is that through the virtue of the *du mai*, all the muscular attachments, especially of the backbone, can be guaranteed to receive the strength of the *qi* and the good irrigation brought by the circulation which is made efficient by the *qi*. If this is not the case there is contraction. Remember the link between the bladder meridian and the *jin*, because at the same level as this point on the bladder meridian is the *shu* point of the liver (Bl 18 *gan yu* 肝俞). So there is a relationship between the function of the *du mai* coupled at this level with the special function of the liver, and the way in which *du mai* can help the liver to master the muscular strength. Of course, muscular strength is a *yang* expression of the body.

Du 9   *zhi yang*   至 陽

Zhi (至) means supreme or absolute, or to reach something; the character contains the image of a bird coming back to its nest at sunset. You can see this from the image of the character with just a little training! It means to reach your goal. All these ideas are contained within this character. The expression *zhi yang* (至 陽) is used in a dual expression with *zhi yin* (至 陰), supreme *yin*, and they are both used frequently in classical texts, for example in Huainanzi chapter 6, which quotes Zhuangzi chapter 21, there is the idea of supreme *yin*, perfect *yin*, black and chilled; and perfect *yang*, supreme *yang*, which burns red and hot. The two mingle and achieve harmony, and from them the ten thousand beings are born.

So why is this point the extreme *yang*? We are concerned with this rising movement and are now at the level of the diaphragm. On the same horizontal line there is the *yu* point of the diaphragm (Bl 17). The diaphragm is here to protect the upper part of the body from unclear influences, it is like a filter, and above the diaphragm we enter the area of the clear *yang*. This is one interpretation of *zhi yang*. We now enter the area of the *yang* which is supreme or perfect. Or possibly, through the *du mai*, we now reach the area of the *yang* which is the part above the diaphragm. And because it is at the level of the diaphragm, it is of course level with the bottom of the lungs, which are related to heaven; they are the master of *qi* and so on. We enter the area of the upper heater which is the residence of the heart.

Another interpretation is that this is the utmost point of the *yang* power, it is like an arch. At the beginning of something there is a lot of tension, and a bursting out – then we reach a summit, a kind of *zhi yang*. But the movement is not yet finished, it is just the middle of the movement, the height, and perhaps this could be the meaning of this point – that we have here the ending of the first part of the rush or push of the vitality from below, and the continuation of the movement to the top of the head.

I'm not sure whether it is possible to make a numerological commentary on the number nine, as it is only number nine according to the modern calculations, and has no meaning in the classical texts. The last point of the bladder meridian is called *zhi yin* (至 陰) and maybe it is because this great *yang* meridian has just reached the *yin*. This is one of the possible interpretations. When it reaches the *yin* it can go no further.

Du 10 *ling tai* 靈 臺

Claude Larre: *Tai* (臺) is a raised terrace and in ancient China people would go to the terraces to be in contact with fresh air, to refresh themselves. The connection with heaven would be so close that the spirits would play around the terraces and enter the mind more easily than at ordinary levels. So it is a place where the spirits are active. This activation of the spirits is called *ling* (靈) in Chinese. *Ling* is one character used to express the effect of the spirits, and that effect is shared with human beings. So *ling tai* gives the idea of an exaltation by the spirits. The character *ling* (靈) is made with the canopy of heaven and four dots representing rain (雨), which is used to express something coming from heaven. Rainfall is always a powerful symbol of a gift from heaven, because this was a time of a primitive agricultural society where people depended on rain to grow crops. Then there is a pictograph of three mouths (口) which represent three sorceresses, as the witchcraft involved in rain making was attributed to women. Below that is the image of two people sitting on the ground.

If we gather all this information together we can see that there is a group of people, sitting on the ground, crying out for heavenly influence. This character soon came to represent the spirits acting for the benefit of humankind. And the activity of the spirits is represented with the character *ming* (明) which is made with the sun and the moon and means brilliance. Because it is made with sun and moon there is an immediate reference to the difference between night and day, and once there is light there is also a way to distinguish things.

So this character *ming* has the meaning of brilliance, and also the ability to distinguish things. When people die they do not remain in nothingness, they return to the indistinct world from which they were taken into life, and in that case to come back to the state of no distinction is also *ming*. The same character is used for the ability to distinguish and to be in the state where there is no longer any distinction. Chinese characters often have this ability to represent one thing and also its opposite.

When we are dealing with the spirits (*shen* 神) we are dealing with our most precious intermediary with heaven. But the special connection between heaven and each individual is that the *shen* come from heaven and dwell in the heart, as long as the heart is tranquil and still. The spirits are always moving around and if they come and stay they change our state of mind, because mind and heart (*xin* 心) are the same character in the Chinese. In order to be in a good relationship with heaven we must offer a very pure heart, and the heart is pure when it is void. So the void in the heart enables us to live at other levels. It is the condition for the spirits to inhabit us. If I am inhabited by the spirits, I will be represented to heaven as someone to care for. The spirits seem to be a necessary intermediary between heaven and my self.

Spirits of this quality should not be confused with the lower level spiritual powers which are not called *shen* but *gui* (鬼). The *gui* are not exactly demons or devils in the Christian sense or even the Buddhist. They are not necessarily such bad guys. They crawl around, remnants of this and that, but they are not totally evil. The devil in the Christian mind is something antagonistic to Christ, which has no relevance in the Chinese or Indian traditions. The *shen* are easy for us to understand, because they are more like angels, but when the *shen* are acting with radiance, the expression in Chinese is *shen ming* (神 明). *Ling* is nearly the same thing as *ming*. It implies some sort of gift of light, which may depend on the authors and the times. In some of the ancient books we have both the expressions *ling tai* (靈 臺), which comes from the Book of Odes, and *shen ming* (神 明).

Elisabeth Rochat: *Ling tai* is also the name of a famous terrace or tower built, according to legend, by King Wen at the beginning of the Zhou dynasty. This terrace was built in a beautiful park where all kinds of animals lived in freedom. And in the Han dynasty, around the time of the beginning of the Christian era, we know that *ling tai* was the name of one of the three ritual buildings of one of the three harmonious halls in the royal palace. These terraces or watchtowers were specially placed so that it was possible see in each direction and also observe the sky, the stars and the constellations.

It was a place for observation, and also for the reception of information, knowledge and spiritual influence; all of that together. It is because the king or the emperor was able to receive this kind of information directly, and because he was able to interpret the information and unify it within himself, that he was considered able to regulate his own life and the life of his people.

For instance, it was because the emperor had good information and knew the exact time and the position of the stars, and whether enemies were approaching or not, he was able to perform the walking ritual within the *ming tang* (明 堂), the house of the calendar. Doing this kind of ritual walking or circum-perambulation around the *ming tang*, he was able to regulate the people in the kingdom and redistribute all the influence he received from above. The *ming tang* was one of the three ritual buildings. *Tang* (堂) is found in the name of Ren 18 (*yu tang* 玉 堂) and it is a temple, or the inner chamber of a building.

In many texts, such as Zhuangzi and many daoist and meditation texts, *ling tai* is the name for the heart, because the heart the sovereign. It must be able to receive information and influence, interpret it correctly and exactly and unify it, in order to be the master of the body.

We can see this in the English translation of a poem from the end of the Han dynasty, which presents the building of a palace:

'The emperor presents the three sacrificial animals, offers the five victims. He worships the celestial and terrestrial spirits (*shen gui* 神 鬼), attracts the hundred deities. He holds audience in the luminous hall (*ming tang* 明 堂) and visits the circular moat. Radiating continuous brightness, he promulgates august teaching. He ascends the divine tower (*ling tai* 靈 臺), studies the good omens, looks up to heaven (*tian* 天) down to the abyss (*kun* 坤), Matching the images to his divine person. Gazing over the Middle Kingdom he dispenses his grace. Viewing the four marches he emanates awesome majesty.'

(Eastern Capital Rhapsody, based on a translation by David R. Knechtges, Princeton University Press).

This is a very good definition of the expression *ling tai*. It is elaborated in the footnote which accompanies the translation.

'The divine tower (*ling tai*) lay slightly south of the luminous hall (*ming tang*). The divine tower served as the imperial observatory, from which the sun, moon, stars, wind, ethers (*qi*), and the pitch pipes were watched.'

In order to be efficient you have to be realistic and you can only be realistic if you know the signs and if you are able to observe reality.

So there are two meanings of *ling tai*. It is the place to observe heaven and receive information and influx coming from above, and consequently it is possible to maintain good order – to maintain regulation and to avoid disorder in the kingdom or in the body. In the body this place is the heart, which is for the reception and the perception of reality and adaptation to reality, too. It is the ability to adapt to the changing outside circumstances. The heart is the dwelling place of the spirits, where we are able to interpret reality and to adapt our conduct. It is in this way that the heart is said, for instance in Suwen chapter 9, to be the place for all change that takes place under the authority of the spirits.

This point is in the area of the heart. Having reached the area of the pure and clear above the diaphragm, the next stage is this possibility for observation, the ability to receive influx, in order to proceed to the *ming tang* (明堂). The next point concerns the ability to conduct one's life according to the information given by the spirits.

Du 11 *shen dao* 神道

The *shen* (神) represent the heavenly inspiration of life, the ability to guide our life. And *dao* (道) is the way, the right way to conduct life according to your innate nature. *Shen dao* is an expression with a very exact meaning. It can be the pathway leading the spirits to the cemetery, the way to turn back towards spirit when we are dealing with worship of the dead. In Japanese *shen dao* is the *shin to* of Shintoism, the way of the spirits. Here on the *du mai* meridian, the most interesting interpretation is of the free communication with the spirits of the heart, which allow the good conduct of life.

And we must not forget that at this level the *du mai* makes a connection between the origin in the lower abdomen and the heart, and that after that it continues to make a connection with the brain and the upper orifices, especially the eyes. It is between these three levels, which we may call the three cinnabar fields (*dan tian* 丹 田), or the dwelling places of the three *hun*, that we also find the three great 'stations' of the *du mai*.

In some old texts of the 3rd and 4th century CE this expression *shen dao* is also the name of a particular section of the magical arts, especially a kind of divinatory art by the observation of the sky, which is a kind of superior integration with the cosmos. We know very little about this kind of magical art, but it is a good expression of *shen dao*, as a kind of conduct which is entirely inspired by the spirits, the total integration of the individual body with the cosmos. And certainly *du mai* has a vital role to play in this integration, through the dynamism of the *yang* between the origin and the heart and the brain. It is a way of communication.

Du 12 *shen zhu* 身柱

It is after this communication with the depths and with the heart and the spirit that there is the possibility for the individual to stand firmly. This character *shen* (身) is often used in the medical texts for the body, but it is also used for an individual person. *Zhu* (柱) is a column, a pillar, and also the name for the column that holds up a house, or a link between heaven and earth. In the old way of representing the square of earth below and the circle of heaven above, they are joined together by eight great pillars. And their name was *zhu*.

The name of Bladder 10 is *tian zhu* (天柱), heavenly pillar, and this is a good place to symbolize the relationship between the head which is like heaven and the body which is like earth. This pillar of Du 12 is not at the neck; anatomically it is level with the central point of the scapula, the great bony mass of the two scapula which reinforces the solidity of the backbone and the ribs. It is at this level that *shen zhu* enables the individual to stand straight like a pillar and ensures communication between above and below.

After the Way of the Spirits, *shen dao*, *shen zhu* is an expression of the free communication with the *qi* and the lungs. This is the level of the *yu* point of the lungs, which gives strength and force to the circulation. There is also this idea of verticality – the ability to stand up straight and the suggestion of a main beam which is taking all the weight of a building. It is very strong, but is also quite vulnerable.

Du 13 *tao dao* 陶 道

Dao (道) is the way, and *tao* (陶) the potter, and also the kiln in which pots are made. It is also a potter's wheel which has a kind of mechanical movement. At the same level at the front of the body is the point *xuan ji* (璇 璣), Ren 21, which suggests something turning and distributing influences. Here on the *du mai* it is the end of the trunk and it suggests the achievement of something, and this is related to the movement of the potter's wheel and the heat of the kiln. That fits quite well with the function of the *du mai* in this area.

If we consider the series of points from Du 9 to Du 13 or 14, this is the area of clear *yang* where it is possible to receive influence and information from heaven (*ling tai),* and from there follow the way inspired by the spirits (*shen dao*). If we follow this way we can achieve the ability to stand up in life (*tian zhu*). Finally something is able to take shape and form – some kind of emanation – and with the movement and heat of *tao dao* something is able to flourish. When this character *tao* (陶) is repeated, *tao tao,* it can mean to be full of elation and joy. It is often used in the Book of Odes in this way. It gives the idea of the celestial *yang* continuing its movement in order to reach the summit of the trunk.

Du 14 *da zhui*   大 椎

Zhui (椎) is a hammer, but the character is also used to refer to the vertebra. This point *da zhui* (大 椎) is located at the top of the back where all the *yang* meridians meet. It is at the base of the neck, the beginning of the passage from the back to the head. This character *zhui* (椎) is made with wood (木) on the left and on the right a character which is used to classify a bunch or a group of things hanging together like a bunch of bananas, or the vertebrae all hanging down and attached to each other. As the final point on the back it is a concentration, a gathering of the *yang*, just before the *du mai* penetrates into the head, the orifices and the brain itself. The next point has a link with the tongue, which also has a direct link to the heart.

Du 15 *ya men* 啞 門

This point is known as *ya men* (啞 門) or *yin men* (瘖 門). *Men* (門) is a gate or a door, as we have seen. *Yin* (瘖) means to be dumb. *Ya* (啞) is also to have difficulty in speaking, and is sometimes translated as hoarseness. The name is explained by the relationship of this point with the tongue. The tongue has a special relationship to the heart and the spirits of the heart, to the formation of words and the ability to speak. If the speech is clear and articulate it is because the *zang*, especially the heart and the liver, are functioning well. If you have some kind of hoarseness, particularly from cold, you need to stimulate the *yang* to resolve the problem. But if it is coming from the depths of the heart or the kidneys it may be some kind of psychological dumbness. Either you can't speak because you have no desire to speak, which is dumbness due to the kidneys, or you don't speak because your mind is not clear enough to organize your speech which is linked with the heart.

It is possible to treat on *du mai* to correct the *yang* of these *zang* and to restore clear speech. It is also possible to work with the power of the lung *qi* for the clarity and power of the voice. So we can see that there is a relationship with the heart and also with the liver for the clear articulation of speech, but also with the kidneys, lungs or spleen, because the essences and *qi* come from the spleen to the other *zang*. This point on the *du mai* is very good to stimulate the *yang* inside the *zang*, to reorganize the speech and resolve dumbness, not only in temporary hoarseness, but for a deeper attack as well.

This is one of the 'nine points to regain the *yang*' given in the classical compendium of acupuncture, the Zhenjiu dacheng, the others are *lao gong* (勞 宮 P 8), *san yin jiao* (三 陰 交 Sp 6), *yong quan* (湧 泉 Ki 1), *tai xi* (太 溪 Ki 3), *zhong wan* (中 脘 Ren 12), *huan tiao* (環 跳 Gb 30), *san li* (三 里 St 36) and *he gu* (合 谷 LI 4).

If there is loss of consciousness, there is a loss of the presence of the spirits and a loss of communication with the exterior. It particularly concerns closure of the upper orifices, and blockage of the communication between the *qi* of the heart and the upper orifices. This point is indicated to restore the *yang* to the upper orifices. Most important is the link with the tongue, and therefore with the speech and the *yang* of the heart.

Du 16 *feng fu* 風 府

This is the storehouse of the wind. As we saw in Nanjing difficulty 28, it is because of its great affinity with the wind and the *yang*, that this point was chosen to express the passage of the *du mai* from the back to the brain. It is also because the *du mai* is the supreme *yang* inside the body, that it has a great power of attraction towards the *yang*, and also with all kinds of *qi* including the wind. This point is at the highest point of the back and it is able to attract the wind – which may be the beneficial *qi* of life, but it could also be perverse wind.

Penetration by wind through *feng fu* is discussed in several classical books, for example in Suwen chapter 35, which presents the progression of a perverse invasion, which starts at *feng fu* and gains ground day after day following the vertebrae, and pushing back the power of the *wei qi*, the defensive *qi*. In other texts there is discussion of perversion and disease inside the brain such as vertigo and also a problem with the eyes coming from perverse penetration through *feng fu*. In Lingshu chapter 33, which gives a presentation of the four seas, *feng fu* is the lower command point for the brain as the sea of marrow. This point is a place of great vitality, and therefore any perverse invasion will be very violent too.

Du 24 *shen ting* 神 庭

Shen (神) is the spirits, *ting* (庭) is a courtyard, a special place inside the ritual architecture of the palace. It is generally just before the entrance to the inner rooms, before the last door, which gives entrance to the emperor's chambers. It is after the great gateway of the entrance and before the door leading to the inner chambers. It is often used as a court of justice. What is important is that it is just before the innermost sacred place and it receives illumination from this inner source. For example, the court of justice of the emperor receives illumination from the emperor's wisdom. It can also provide a place to observe visitors and decide whether to see them or not.

Shen ting is a place of reception and observation, with an enlightenment coming from the spirits for the brain and the eyes, taking advantage of the clear essences coming from the five *fu* and rising to the level of the eyes and the brain. At this level of the front of the forehead, we can see the expression of the relationship between the *du mai* and the heart, and the power of the spirits in the brain, because the brain is sometimes called the palace or the storehouse for the *yuan shen* (元 神), the spirits which are from the origin. The presence of the spirits inside the brain is essential and this is a place where the spirits are not in their dwelling place, which is the heart. On the *ren mai* for example, in the area of the heart, there is a different kind of courtyard with the point *yu tang* (玉 堂). But *shen ting* is a courtyard where the spirits can practise their enlightenment and give out their light, not completely hidden but protected by the bone of the skull, as the spirits of the heart are protected by the canopy of the lung.

Du 26 *shui gou* 水溝

Shui (水) is water, *gou* (溝) a kind of ditch. It is a description of the nasal labial groove. This groove is between the nose and the mouth, between the two upper orifices which have a special relationship with *du mai*. The nose is for receiving the *qi* of heaven through the breath, the mouth for receiving the *qi* of earth coming from food. This groove is just between heaven and earth in the upper orifices, a place for the reception of *qi* and essences. In physiognomy, this groove is seen as the centre of all the orifices, because above there are the three *yang* orifices, the nose, eyes and ears, and below the three *yin* orifices, the mouth and the two lower orifices. That is just one way of looking at the central position of this point – between *yin* and *yang*, between heaven and earth, between *qi* and essences (*jing* 精). That is the reason why it is also called *ren zhong* (人 中) meaning the centre of the being.

It is also very close to the meeting with the *ren mai* and, especially in the Neijing, these last points of *du mai*, 27 and 28, sometimes belong to *ren mai*, it is not always clear. This is the area of the connection between the *yin* and the *yang* through the *du mai* and *ren mai*. There is also a relationship with the *yang ming* meridians, the stomach and large intestine. The stomach is of course also linked to the centre, the earth, and the meridian has a central position.

But this may also be a reference to the kind of exercise given in daoist books in which to nourish the vital principle you close the mouth, touch the tongue against the upper palate and swallow the liquids and saliva which accumulate in the mouth. This allows them to irrigate and humidify the whole organism and to increase the strength of the *zang* and the *fu*, and all the bone articulations, by the quality of the essences which enrich themselves with the preservation and the swallowing of body fluids (*jin ye* 津 液) and saliva.

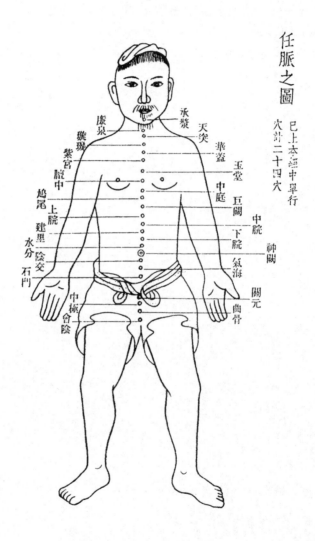

Ren mai from the Neiwaigong tushuo

REN MAI 任 脈

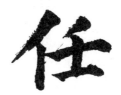

Elisabeth Rochat: The study of *ren mai* itself will be quite short as some of the functions are best studied with *chong mai*. But first let us look at the character *ren* (任). It is composed with the radical *ren* (人), human, and the phonetic (壬) which is found in Wieger Lesson 82 C, and is etymologically speaking an image of a bamboo pole with a load hanging at each end, buckets of water for example. The meaning is to endure, to bear, to take the burden of something. When you add the radical for the human being (任) it becomes to bear the burden of being human, which is for instance, to be able to take charge and cope at each level of human life: to cope with each situation, to endure, to withstand, and to be able to resist attack. At the same time, this idea of being able to withstand is softened by the notion of following the natural way. It is to cope, not by confrontation, but allowing. The character also has the meaning to be worthy of confidence and full of sincerity, to be reliable.

The phonetic part (壬) is the character of the ninth of the ten celestial stems and suggests something acting in the depths but not manifesting itself. The tenth celestial stem is *gui* (癸) which is the secret movement of waters in the depths of the earth, and is also the character used in the expression designating human fertility (*tian gui* 天 癸), as we see in Suwen chapter 1, where *ren mai* and *chong mai* are in charge of producing fertility in women. If we add to the phonetic part the character for woman (女) we have *ren* (妊), a pregnant woman, or to be with child. And remember that when we added the character woman to the character *du* (叔), it gave the meaning of the woman in charge of all the women in the palace, a kind of governess. Adding the radical of the silk thread, the meaning is to weave, *ren* (紝).

The relationship with pregnancy is of course significant, and in the classical commentaries the *ren mai* is related to pregnancy. This is the meridian which acts to nourish life; it provides all the essences, blood and fluids to nourish the new life inside a woman's body. But of course *ren mai* does not exist only in women, or only in a pregnant woman, but it acts in the same way at all times for all people; it provides all the elements to nourish life, not only a new life growing within me, but also for my own life. And that is the meaning of *ren*; to be able to endure and to continue, and to continuously ensure the nourishing of life.

The function of *ren mai* is to command and control all the *yin* functions within the body. *Ren mai* is called the sea of the *yin* meridians and the special master for the uterus and the function of gestation inside a woman. All kinds of enveloping and protecting and bringing together of the elements of life constitute the *yin* aspect of vitality, and are under the authority of *ren mai*. This must be the reason why *ren mai* is sometimes translated as 'conception vessel', and sometimes as 'controller vessel'. Conception is too narrow a translation, as conception is only one aspect of the function of the *ren mai*, but through the Chinese character we can understand the link between these two ideas. It is not only the conception of a new life, but the nourishment of this new life and the nourishment of each individual life, with the same regulation and the same protection that is given to the embryo. *Ren mai* is also the controller, because it is able to master and control all the *yin* within the body.

THE PATHWAY OF REN MAI

Elisabeth Rochat: The pathway of *ren mai* is not so strange and complicated as *du mai*. The pattern is given in Nanjing difficulty 28:

> '*Ren mai* arises below the central pole (*zhong ji* 中 極, Ren 2) and rises to the border of the (pubic) hair; it passes along the abdomen on the inside; it rises to *guan yuan* (關 元 Ren 4); it reaches the throat (*hou yan* 喉 咽, larynx and pharynx).'

We have seen that *du mai* begins its circulation at this inner injection of vitality called the inferior pole, and that this may refer to Ren 1, *hui yin* (會 陰). Below *zhong ji* (中 極), the central pole, is perhaps another way to designate the same point. *Zhong ji* is the name of Ren 3, but this is not the starting point of the meridian, because the text says 'below the central pole', the centre in the depths of the lower abdomen, which is the centre of the beginning of life. It could also be said to begin at the same place as *du mai*, at *hui yin*, Ren 1. Some commentators suggest that it begins at Ren 2, others say that it begins at Du 1, to emphasize the crossing effect of *ren* and *du mai*, and the interpenetration of *yin* and *yang* in the beginning.

Ren mai then turns to the interior. Again only one point is indicated: *guan yuan* (關 元 Ren 4) and again the choice is quite symbolic. It is chosen because *guan yuan* is below the navel in this area of great *yin* activity in the lower heater, and *guan yuan* (關 元 The Passage to the Origin) expresses the function of *ren mai* very well: it means to remain in connection with the origin, and through this connection to give the exact, authentic and primitive rule to all the *yin* functioning within the body. At the same time, it is the ability to nourish a new life which originates there.

Compared to *feng fu* (風 府), which turns towards the exterior at the top of the body and is related to the wind, the *qi* and movement, *guan yuan* (關 元) turns towards the interior and to the origin. The *du mai* continues through *feng fu* to the brain, the *ren mai* continues to reach the throat. The throat is the passage for all the *yin* fluids between the body and the head. All the meridians in this area, and particularly the kidney meridian, raise fluids to the upper orifices. And points on the *ren mai* such as Ren 18, 22 and 23 are very important for regulating the fluids ascending inside the body.

The throat is also a passage for food to descend to the stomach for the assimilation of essences. The throat is an important place for the meeting of the *yin* meridians; it is also mentioned in the description of the *yin qiao mai* in the same chapter of the Nanjing, making a connection with *ren mai* and *chong mai*.

So here we have the first kind of opposition of a couple of points, one on the back for the *yang* and one on the abdomen for the *yin*, and within the opposition the idea of the *yang* function and the *yin* function. For *feng fu*, the animation of the *yang*, and for *guan yuan*, how to build and nourish life with all the *yin* elements of blood and fluids. The *yang* and the *qi* are associated with 'no form', but the *yin*, the blood and the construction of a new life and the renewal of life are concerned with shape and form. This is also a comparison made by some commentators: the *yang* is formless but the *yin* has form and is concerned with the construction of the physical form.

But there is always a crossing effect. The *du mai*, even if it is in charge of the *yang* and the *qi*, needs to have a very strong relationship with the *yin*, especially with the *yin* of the kidneys, the authentic *yin*, original water and so on. *Ren mai*, which is in charge of the blood and the *yin*, to nourish the body and the form, has a connection not only with original water but also with original *yang* or fire.

The two 'seas of *qi*' are on the *ren mai*, one at Ren 6 (*qi hai* 氣 海) which is the connection with the original *qi*, and the other at Ren 17 (*tan zhong* 膻 中) the sea of *qi* in the centre of the chest. To the Chinese way of thinking it is normal to to have this kind of combined penetration and mixing of *yin* and *yang*. Nothing can exist which is only *yin* or only *yang*; the *yin* can only circulate with the *yang* and the *yang* can only be effective with the *yin*. All the commentators emphasize the meeting of water and fire, *qi* and blood for *ren* and *du mai*, and always in relation to this kind of mixing and crossing.

Suwen chapter 60:

> '*Ren mai* arises below the central pole, *zhong ji* (中 極), and rises to the border of the (pubic) hair; it passes through the abdomen on the inside; it rises to *guan yuan* (關 元); it reaches the throat, (*hou yan* 喉 咽, larynx and pharynx), rises to the chin, passes through the face and penetrates the eyes.'

Suwen chapter 60 provides another way to look at this interpenetration and relationship between the *yin* and the *yang*. It gives exactly the same description as in the Nanjing, but the trajectory continues up to the eyes, which are also a meeting point with the *du mai*, allowing the *yin* to join the *yang* at the top of the body in order to nourish the uppermost orifices and the brain.

Lingshu chapter 65:

> '*Chong mai* and *ren mai* both arise in the middle of the intimate envelopes (*bao zhong* 胞 中); they rise, running up the back on the inside and make the sea of the *jing*

luo (經 絡). Their pathway emerges and runs along the abdomen by the right and rises. They meet together at the pharynx; a divergence (*bie* 別) takes a *luo* (絡) relationship with the lips and the mouth.'

We will look at this pathway later with *chong mai*, but it is important to complete our understanding by looking at this view of the *ren mai*. Here *ren mai* gives a kind of support to the backbone from its origin in the intimate envelope of vitality. The common origin of *du mai*, *ren mai*, and *chong mai* is in this area *bao zhong* (胞 中), the area of the hidden origin where, according to Nanjing difficulty 39, it is possible to draw from life what is necessary to make another life. The extraordinary vessels which are so important for the building of my own life are also important for the building of a new life, because it is this same location, the same function and the same richness that is at work.

Ren mai and *du mai* begin together, and then *ren mai* just rises, passing by the Horizontal Bone, Ren 2, which also has an alternative name with the meaning of a maze, a maze leading to a hidden and secret place. Ren 3, *zhong ji*, is the Ridge Pole, the centre of life in the depths of the vitality, and then *guan yuan* (關 元 Ren 4) is the Passage to the Origin. After these points comes Ren 6, the Sea of Qi (*qi hai* 氣 海). At Ren 7 (*yin qiao* 陰 交) there is the idea of exchange, not only within the *yin* but also an exchange between *yin* and *yang* at this level of the origin and the constitution of the body, with this meeting just below the navel.

The following points, Ren 10, 12 and 13 have a very strong

connection with the stomach. The stomach is very important in the Neijing for the renewal of the body for both the *yin* and *yang*. *Ren mai* and *chong mai* have a very strong relationship not only with the kidneys and pre-heaven, but also with the stomach and post-heaven for the renewal of vitality.

The progression of the points on the chest suggests a kind of protection for the heart and the upper heater. Some points, like the Purple Palace (*zi gong* 紫宮, Ren 19) not only refer to the heart, but also to the colour of the blood, and *tan zhong* (膻中 Ren 17), the Sea of Qi in the middle of the chest, evokes all the circulation of blood and *qi* in the chest and all the messengers and ministers and servants obeying the heart.

If *ren mai* is in charge of controlling the blood and gives the rules for the circulation and renewal of the blood and other *yin* functions of the body, then it has to have a relationship with the heart, because the heart is the place where blood becomes blood. It is also the place, with all the other functions of the upper heater, where the circulation of blood is mastered and ruled. In all kinds of pathology linked to the circulation of blood, especially for women, it is not only a question of the relationship between *ren mai* and *chong mai* and kidneys, liver and spleen, but also with the heart.

Then there is a Passage to Heaven (*tian tu* 天突, Ren 22), which is like a chimney, a passage leading to the head and to heaven. And in the case of *ren mai* it is a passage for the circulation of fluids, not only the blood but all the fluids of the organism which pass through the throat. Finally at the eyes and at the lips there is a connection with the *du mai*, closing the cycle and providing continuous exchange and circulation.

The *du mai* and the *ren mai* have a common origin, then there is divergence and differentiation before they meet again at another level. It is a manifestation of vitality which always remains connected with its origin, but expresses itself in the adult and responsible human as the ability to guide his or her own life. The *yang* and the spirits permeate the whole body, and are stored in the interior; all the substances required for the vitality of the body are supplied through the regular mastering of the *yin* function.

This is one of the great functions of the extraordinary meridians, especially the first four, *du mai, ren mai, chong mai* and *dai mai* – to preserve and ensure the link of all the diverse *yin* and *yang* functions in the body with the origin.

We have not covered the meeting of *ren mai* and *du mai* with the other meridians, but that can be found easily in other books. At the level of the throat, the connection with the kidney meridian is quite strong and below the centre of the eyes and at the lips the connection with the stomach meridian is also strong.

Claude Larre: Since there are two systems, a primary system with *du mai, ren mai, chong mai* and *dai mai*, and so on, and a secondary system, it is important to see where there is a relationship between them. One of the most important things about this teaching is the understanding of relationships. If one meridian follows another, or crosses with another, the difficulty is not in the relationship but in the selection of the places where this relationship is observed. Because when touching this particular point in treatment, you will have a more specific effect, bringing in the specific attributes of the twelve main meridians but also accessing the eight. Understanding where these two systems interact is very important in practice, because one is the primary and the other the secondary. And where they touch each other they are the same thing. The point has a particular function which encompasses the properties of both systems.

This is not an academic view, but a practical understanding of how life functions – because it has been organized by the primary system and developed by the secondary one.

Question: I have been noticing as we go on that Bladder 1 (*jing ming* 睛 明) seems to be assuming more importance.

Elisabeth Rochat: Yes, of course, and it is also a meeting point for the *qiao mai*. It is a point that has so many interconnections. Its name evokes so many things, for example the luminous radiance of the eyes which comes from essences impregnated by the spirits. According to Suwen chapter 81, or Lingshu 80, there is a gathering of the purest essences of the five *zang* and six *fu* at the eyes. *Ming* (明) describes this kind of luminous radiance, and *jing* (睛) is the pupil. The character is made with the eye (目) and the phonetic *jing* (青) which suggests the vibrant green colour of nature but also forms part of the character for clear and pure (*qing* 清) and for essences (*jing* 精).

In Lingshu 17, for example, we see that all these pathways and crossings (not only *ren mai*, *du mai*, and *qiao mai*, but all the *yang* meridians passing around the eyes and the brain, and the pathways of the *yin* meridians of the heart and liver too) ensure the clarity and purity of the sight externally, the clarity and purity of the heart within, as well as the ability to perceive things correctly. The eyes also have the ability to ensure the correct rhythm of life, adapting to the regularity of the rising and setting of the sun, and adapting to the seasons.

One of the meanings of this meeting is the brightness of the eyes and the enlightenment of our whole perception. The eyes are what we present to others, because, according to Zhuangzi and other authors, it is through the pupil of the eyes that we can see the depths of a person. That is not exactly an answer to your question, but this all comes into play.

Claude Larre: It would be interesting to select the points which are obviously very active in this way and to see how the twelve main meridians give the specific functions and the extraordinary meridians the more general. Because life at the origin is more chaotic, and becomes much more organized and elaborate as life progresses. There are so many places where life interacts in this way, and if we can begin to see the correspondences between these processes we may come closer to an understanding of life at its origin. Then we will be able to call on life at the deeper level in order to remedy some defect or the other. We work on the general system of twelve, but we also call on the deeper sources of life. So the question could be treated theoretically, but whenever you have a good result it may be that you are using points where the purest essences are available.

Comment: Another idea would be that the effects of the extraordinary meridians are so much deeper and homogeneous and profound and primitive and so close to the edge of human understanding that as we have a list of World Health Organization approved points to use, one must have a list of points to avoid, because we have non-intervention based on the difficulty to understand.

Claude Larre: It could be that the ones that are forbidden are the ones to use – because they are powerful. But not to be used by just anybody.

PATHOLOGY OF REN MAI

Nanjing difficulty 29:

> 'When *ren mai* gives rise to illness, one suffers by being knotted internally (*nei jie* 內 結). In men this gives the seven *shan* (*qi shan* 七 疝) and in women concretions and accumulations (*jia ju* 瘕 聚).'

Suwen chapter 60:

> 'When *ren mai* gives rise to illness, in men there is knotting internally (*nei jie* 內 結) and there are the seven *shan* (*qi*

shan 七 疝); in women there are discharges (*dai xia* 帶 下) as well as concretions and accumulations (*jia ju* 瘕 聚).'

Elisabeth Rochat: The most important thing with these pathologies is an exaggeration of the *yin* movement. A knot or an accumulation is an exaggeration of the movement of condensation and accumulation leading to a piling up and the formation of some kind of clot or lump internally. If something is flowing out in the form of a discharge, especially vaginal discharge, it is in the form of fluid or a perversion of fluids. Vaginal discharge (*dai xia* 帶 下) is also governed by *dai mai*. It is the same character (*dai* 帶) that is used in both.

'Internal knotting' emphasizes the function of *ren mai* to regulate the circulation of blood and fluids in the lower abdomen, and to nourish all the functions of the inner abdomen. If it does not do that, there may be some kind of knotting in the inner part of the abdomen. This is very often due to cold or emptiness of *qi* leading to blockage and congestion in the circulation and distribution of blood and all the elements necessary for life. This is the reason why there are these accumulations which may be clots and lumps of any kind.

There are two words (*jia* 瘕 and *ju* 聚) used for this kind of accumulation. *Jia* are quite fixed and hard, and when palpated they do not move; *ju* may move on palpation. Here *jia ju* relates to any kind of concentration and accumulation in the lower heater and the abdomen. In the case of *jia*, we would definitely expect something physical and solid, with *ju* not necessarily, but they are very general terms.

As *ren mai* has responsibility for the *yin* part of the body, it also has the responsibility to ensure free circulation in the *yin* part of the body and for the *yin* in general. For example, in the lower heater the *ren mai* has a strong connection with the three *yin* meridians of the legs, the liver, kidneys and spleen; they can be treated at Ren 3 or at the meeting of the three leg *yin* at Spleen 6 (*san yin jiao* 三 陰 交) to invigorate the circulation in the lower heater. It is possible to treat on the *ren mai* or on the *yin* meridians in order to do that.

Here the pathology of *ren mai* includes all kinds of stagnation and weakness of the circulation in the lower heater, leading to knots and accumulations, but we can also see the importance of the warmth of *qi* and *yang*. If the *qi* is deficient the *ren mai* cannot be in balance. Emptiness, weakness and cold invade this area and cause congestion and blockage, especially causing the symptoms called *shan* (疝), which is sometimes translated as hernia, but actually includes all kinds of symptoms of the lower abdomen. There may be pain, which is sometimes quite violent, but there may also be disturbance in the two lower orifices or the genitals. All those conditions may be called *shan*.

It is possible to divide these *shan* syndromes into three categories: those of hernia, those of pain in the lower abdomen and those of the genitals and two lower orifices. They are linked with *ren mai* because they are all symptoms of the lower abdomen and are usually caused by a lack of circulation, quite often due to cold. This term *shan* is very broad and can be used for other symptoms, not only the seven *shan* commonly attributed to the malfunction of *ren mai*. There are also *shan* due to heat and dampness, but particularly in the genitals or testicles it is often due to cold. Wind may cause *shan* syndromes too. The seven *shan* are described slightly differently by different commentators but the most common description is of *han shan* (寒 疝, cold *shan*), *shui shan* (水 疝, water *shan*), *jin shan* (筋 疝, muscle *shan*), *xue shan* (血 疝, blood *shan*), *qi shan* (氣 疝), *hu shan* (狐 疝, fox *shan*) and *tui shan* (㿉 疝, *shan* of the genitals).

Du mai also circulates in this area, and *shan* syndrome appears in the pathology of *du mai*, in common with *ren mai* and *chong mai*, with symptoms not only of the lower orifices but also of the heart, because the counter-current caused by obstruction in the lower abdomen can create pressure of *qi* under the heart.

The pathology of *ren mai*, with *chong mai* and *du mai* too, is connected with women's fertility and all kinds of problems concerned with gynaecology and obstetrics; the regulation of menstruation, sterility and menopause and so on. In Suwen chapter 1 we have the following:

'...In a woman of two times seven years, fertility (*tian gui* 天 癸) arrives; *ren mai* functions fully (*tong* 通) and *tai chong mai* (太 衝 脈, the powerful *chong mai*) rises in power (*sheng* 盛); the menses flow downwards in their time and she has children...'

'...At seven times seven years, the *ren mai* is empty (*xu* 虛) the *tai chong mai* declines progressively, fertility dries up. Nothing passes any longer through the way of earth (*di dao* 地 道); the body declines, and she no longer has children.'

This is the normal cycle for women, but if the *ren mai* becomes empty before its time there is a closing of the 'way of earth'. The way of the earth may be used to designate the vagina, but it can also refer to all the functions of a woman's body which reflect the properties of the earth, which of course are more active in women, such as the ability to receive and to condense, to keep firm, and to nourish – which is all important for fertility in women. For men fertility is more concerned with seminal emissions.

So for women, *ren mai* is the basis of this kind of earthly movement, through its natural function of mastering the *yin*. If the *ren mai* is too weak, then the function of receiving and the ability to nourish and protect, to condense and to keep, is too weak, and that is one cause of sterility. The various causes and different kinds of sterility may be linked with different meridians, for example the *yin* meridians of the foot, particularly the kidneys and the liver, but also the spleen and heart.

The following are some common symptoms for the *ren mai* in classical texts:

'...movement like a beating, with acute hard pain in the lower abdomen, especially around the navel, and with radiation from the navel to the symphisis pubis.'

'...all kinds of hard pain in the region of the genitals, as we saw with the *shan* syndromes.'

'...pain in the abdomen 'like a finger' which has a regular movement and affects the heart.'

'...inability to bend down or to stand up, due to a weakness in the *ren mai*, with a lack of moistening, lack of fluids and blood, leading to a kind of congestion of *qi* and stiffness of the body.'

Ren mai and the points on the *ren mai* meridian are very important in the treatment of women, but if there is a problem with the genitals and sexual organs in men, *ren mai* should be treated as well as *du mai*. In impotence, spermatorrhoea or premature ejaculation, the diagnosis would often suggest treatment on both *ren mai* and *du mai*. *Ren mai* is also very important in the treatment of miscarriage, because it is the power of the *yin* to contain and retain, and to envelop and keep.

Question: What about the relationship of *ren mai* with the upper and middle heaters?

Elisabeth Rochat: That comes more with the command points and with the connection with *yin wei mai*. But we can use points on the *ren mai* for many other things. We have been talking about the symptoms particularly linked to a weakness in the functioning of *ren mai*, and these symptoms are always in the lower heater and to do with the production and reproduction of the innermost elements of life, maintaining a good rhythm for their regulation and distribution.

But of course we can use the points on *ren mai* in many different ways. If there is a problem with the stomach we may use the points of *ren mai* at this level, and in its function of mastering the *yin, ren mai* has a relationship with the root of the essences of post-heaven and the distribution of all the elements of life, as well as the constitution and circulation of the blood. *Tan zhong* (膻 中), Ren 17, has this function.

We must not confuse the indications of all the points of *ren mai* and *du mai* with the main symptoms at the root of the functioning of *ren mai* and *du mai*. For *du mai* the characteristic of these symptoms is this kind of stiffness, which is a lack of suppleness in the verticality of the body and a lack of the circulation which provides animation and dynamism, especially to the head. With *ren mai* there is a kind of excessive condensation and concentration in the lower part of the trunk.

Question: Some teachings say that one should not mix the treatment of the extraordinary meridians with other points. Is there any reference in the classics to that?

Elisabeth Rochat: There is always contradiction in the teachings of different schools, within China as well as in the West. It is similar to the question asked previously on the forbidden points. And it depends on what you call the classics. I am sure you will find it somewhere, but I have no answer to your question. I think it may be part of the teaching of some special schools, and sometimes things are really forbidden, but often it is just advising that you must know what you are doing. This is certainly not a general teaching.

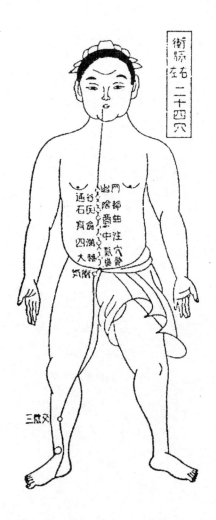

Chong mai from the Neiwaigong tushuo

CHONG MAI 衝 脈

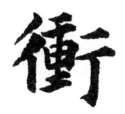

Elisabeth Rochat: The character *chong* (衝) is made up of two parts; the first is the radical (*xing* 行), which is split and can be seen on the left and right sides of the character. It means to walk well, and is a repetition of the same thing. As we can see in the etymology in Wieger lesson 63 C, it is to take a step forward with the left foot – putting the left foot forward and finishing the step with the right.

One of the early meanings of *xing* is to march, and also to circulate; it is a circulation that is without fault and error, flowing effortlessly from one stage to another; it is also a pattern or model for good circulation and exchange. Of course this is the character used for the five elements or five phases (*wu xing* 五 行). Here the meaning of the radical is motion or circulation.

The phonetic *chong* (重) appears between the two parts of the radical. In Wieger lesson 120 K this character is explained as a human being (人) on the top, trying to raise from the earth (土) at the bottom, an object which is seen at the centre. The earliest meaning of the character is to be heavy; it is a heavy weight or a great effort. A second is the repetition of an effort. The third meaning is of something serious, for example a serious illness; serious because it is very important and essential. The ideogram is the image of an accumulation. The idea of power and the effort to raise something is very strong in the early meanings of this character *chong*.

The most common interpretation of *chong* (衝) is of a great route of communication, a route with a lot of crossings or tributaries. And as people are able to meet together because of this major route, then the main idea of *chong* is not just the meeting of routes but also the ability to continue straight ahead, gathering more and more things on the way from the other routes that join.

One common meaning of this character *chong* is to go straight ahead. It suggests a very important route, a very important passage, and sometimes a strategic route – but it also implies that the movement and circulation facilitated by such a route is quite fast and quick. You can drive much faster on a motorway than on a small country road, and you can show the power of your car. The character also suggests the idea of a rush, a push. In military vocabulary it is to attack with great strength and impetuosity and it is used in a term for a special kind of battering ram. It is something full of vigour and power.

If we add the radical of the ear of corn (種) to the phonetic it gives the idea of a seed and to sow. In the seed there is a concentration of power able to break out and push up through the earth. Adding the radical for the body (腫) the character becomes one of many characters used to describe a pregnant woman. With the image of a tendon (*dong* 動), it is the character used to express the movement of life, for example the beating of the heart. The term for zoology, the science of living things, is made with this character. With the radical for vegetation it means to regulate, to govern, to overlook, to administrate (*dong*, 董).

These related characters can help us to understand the implied meaning of *chong*. It is a great power, the power of the seed of life and the promise of life, animated with the vigour of the movement of life and the living being. It is very important and serious and is able to regulate and administer something. Sometimes commentators emphasize the rapidity, and they explain *chong* as the way to ensure that all circulation is quick and correct.

So why is *chong mai* so important? All the texts, especially the Neijing, stress the fact that the *chong mai* is able to regulate both blood and *qi*. Because of that *chong mai* is called the 'sea of blood', but it is also called the 'sea of the meridians'. And of course the meridians are nothing but the regulation of the circulation of *qi*, allowing the blood and *qi* to circulate in the correct way without deviation.

THE PATHWAY OF CHONG MAI

Nanjing difficulty 28:

> '*Chong mai* arises at *qi chong* (氣 衝 St 30) the crossroads of the *qi*; it doubles the pathway of the *yang ming* of the foot (the stomach meridian); it surrounds the navel and rises. It reaches the middle of the thorax (*xiong zhong* 胸 中) and diffuses there.'

We can add the description in Suwen 60:

> '*Chong mai* arises at the street of *qi* (*qi jie* 氣 街); doubling the pathway of the *shao yin* (the kidney meridian) it surrounds the navel and rises; it reaches the middle of the thorax (*xiong zhong* 胸 中) and diffuses there.'

The pathway is very similar in the Suwen and the Nanjing, but one has the *chong mai* doubling the *yang ming* of the foot (stomach meridian), the other the *shao yin* of the foot (kidney meridian). This is a short trajectory rising from the bottom of the abdomen, not in the centre but at both sides, at *qi chong* (St 30). The name *qi chong* (氣 衝) is made from the character for *qi* (氣) and the same character *chong* (衝) that we find in *chong mai*: 'vigorous street of *qi*'. This is not exactly the beginning or origin of *chong mai*, but it is the starting point of its pathway on the front of the body, which passes through the navel, or close to the navel, to the area of the sea of *qi* in the centre of the chest, with a movement of effusion and expansion in the upper heater.

The most important thing about this trajectory is the power of the movement of *qi* coming from the point of emergence in the lower abdomen. At the level of the chest the *qi* is a unification of the *qi* of the stomach and the *qi* from the lower heater, which comes up through the navel to the sea of *qi* at the centre of the chest and regulates its circulation throughout the whole body. Through the ancestral *qi*, or *zong qi* (宗 氣), the *qi* is given the principle of leadership and unified mastership to guide it into the regular circulation of the defensive and nutritive *qi*, and to guide the rhythmic circulation through the twelve meridians.

The the function of the lungs, the sea of *qi* and the heart, is to regulate the 100 *mai*. The 100 *mai* represent the whole network of animation and circulation throughout the body, meridians as well as all other connections and networks of relationships and circulations, even the smallest and most superficial. This is the first function of *chong mai*. *Chong mai* is concerned with *qi*, and with creating a good rhythm of circulation. It makes the connection between the sea of *qi* at the origin and the sea of *qi* in the chest.

In other texts *chong mai* is given other trajectories and other functions. And often the trajectories are actually symbolic of the function. For example in Lingshu 38:

> The *chong mai* is the sea of the five *zang* and six *fu*. Its rising part emerges from the nasopharynx, filters into all the *yang*, irrigates all the essences.

> Its descending part pours out into the great *luo* of the

shao yin, arises under the kidneys, leaves the street of *qi* (*qi jie* 氣 街), runs along the internal face of the *yin* aspect of the thigh; obliquely penetrates the middle of the back of the knee, buries itself and circulates on the internal face of the tibia; together with the *shao yin* meridian it descends and penetrates behind the medial malleolus; it penetrates under the foot.

'Its detachment (*bie* 別) together with the *shao yin*, filters into the three *yin*, obliquely penetrates the malleolus, buries itself and circulates, leaves and takes a dependent relation with the top of the foot, penetrates between the big toe; it filters into all the *luo* (絡) and warms the flesh of the foot and the leg.'

Through its ascending movement the *chong mai* reaches its highest point – the inner orifices of the nose and the area between the nose and mouth – just at the level of the contact between heaven and earth. The mouth is the orifice of earth, the nose the orifice for heaven, as have seen. *Chong mai*, being linked with the *qi* and the blood, is connected with both the *qi* of heaven and the essences coming from earth. We can see the connecting movement of *chong mai*, making bridges, bringing together the two facets of reality, heaven and earth, *yin* and *yang*, *qi* and blood. Because at its highest level *chong mai* is in the area of the *yang*, it is able to filter into the *yang* and penetrate all the *yang* circulation. *Chong mai* is like the mother of the *yang* circulation, it provides the *yang* with essences, fluids and blood, which enable the *yang* to be efficient.

After that there is a description of a descending trajectory which makes a strong link with *shao yin* of the foot, the kidney meridian, or the *luo* of the kidney meridian. It runs to the knee, descending the internal face of the tibia to the internal malleolus, finally penetrating underneath the foot, which suggests the first point of the kidney meridian, *yong quan* (湧 泉). Another name for this point is *di chong* (地 衝). *Di* (地) is the earth, with the *chong* (衝) of *chong mai*, and it means that the power of the *chong mai* joins with the power of the earth at this point. After that there is a kind of delegation of power – the power of *chong mai* has joined with the power of the earth, which enables it to filter into the *yin* circulation.

Then the text describes a pathway penetrating the top of the foot and the inside of the big toe, which suggests a link with all three *yin* meridians of the foot and the stomach meridian. That it 'filters into the *luo*' suggests that it is not only the main meridians which are concerned here but that the action of *chong mai* is felt in the network of the more superficial and more detailed circulation too – penetrating the mass of the body, warming the flesh of the feet and the legs. This implies the *yang* power of the *qi*, because the *qi* warms the flesh, especially through the circulation of the *luo*. So the *chong mai* has a kind of mastery of the *yang* circulation, at the same time enriching the *qi* with essences. But it also masters the *yin* circulation, bringing warmth, heat and movement into the territory covered by the *yin* circulation. That is the reason why the *chong mai* is said to be 'the sea of the twelve meridians'.

We have seen that *du mai* has a special mastery of the *yang* meridians and the *yang* function throughout the body, and *ren mai* has the same for the *yin*. Now in the third position *chong mai* is able to gather and inter-penetrate these two powers. The text of Lingshu chapter 38 shows this double aspect of vitality through the pathway of the *chong mai*. At the beginning of the text *chong mai* is not called 'the sea of the meridians', but 'the sea of the five *zang* and six *fu*'.

This text gives us a complete presentation of the *chong mai*. If it is beneath and behind the *yin* as well as the *yang* circulation, and behind the essences as well as the ability to warm, it is able to master all the various kinds of circulation and the balance between *yin* and *yang*, between essences, blood and *qi*, and is able to provide a pattern of vitality for the five *zang* and six *fu*. That is the reason why it is the sea of the five *zang* and six *fu*.

It shares this name with the stomach, which is also said to be the sea of the five *zang* and six *fu*, because the stomach is in charge of the renewal of essences and *qi*. We can see here the strong relationship between the *chong mai* and the stomach meridian, which work together. The stomach continually renews the essences through digestion and assimilation, but it is unable to regulate the distribution of *qi* and essences on its own. The *chong mai* represents the pattern of organization for this distribution.

In Lingshu chapter 62 the *chong mai* is presented as the 'sea of the twelve meridians':

'The *chong mai* is the sea of the twelve meridians (*jing* 經). With the great *luo* of the *shao yin*, it arises under the kidneys and leaves at the street of *qi* (*qi jie* 氣 街) St 30. It runs along the upper part of the internal aspect of the thigh and obliquely penetrates the middle of the popliteal crease; it runs along the leg inside together with the meridian of *shao yin*; it descends and penetrates behind the internal malleolus; it penetrates underneath the foot.'

This is almost the same as chapter 38, but two things are added. One is the starting point, which is given as below the kidneys; *qi chong* is the point where the power of the *qi* emerges.

Lingshu chapter 65:

'*Chong mai* and *ren mai* both arise in the middle of the intimate envelopes (*bao zhong* 胞 中); they rise up the back on the inside and make the sea of the *jing luo* (經 絡). Their pathway, emerged and external, runs along the abdomen to the right and then rises. They meet together at the pharynx; a divergence (*bie* 別) takes a *luo* (絡) relation with the lips and the mouth.'

Here the starting point is not just below the kidneys but in the middle of the envelope of vitality. The pathway is much the same, but we will come back to this a bit later.

Suwen chapter 44:

'The *yang ming* is the sea of the five *zang* and six *fu*.

It commands the humidification of the ancestral muscle (*zong jin* 宗筋). The ancestral muscle commands the bony chain; it gives ease to the mechanism of the other articulations (*ji guan* 機關).'

If there is a place for mastery of all the muscular forces, and if the mass of the muscles are attached to the bone, then all the interplay of the bone articulations depends not only on a good irrigation, but also on the strength and suppleness of the attachment of the muscles to the bones. This is the reason why the *zong jin* (宗筋), the so-called ancestral muscle, which is the common place for all the muscular forces throughout the body, is in charge of the articulation of the spine. Suwen chapter 44 continues:

'*Chong mai* is the sea of the *jing mai* (經脈). It commands humidification and irrigation through impregnation of the small and large valleys (*xi gu* 谿谷). It makes its junction (*he* 合) with the *yang ming* at the ancestral muscle.'

There is another mention here of the relationship between *chong mai* and the *yang ming* of the foot, the stomach meridian, concerning the control of movement throughout the body. This movement depends on the muscular forces and the irrigation of all the parts of the body. If there is dryness in any articulation, in the bones and the muscles and flesh, movement will become more and more difficult and stiffness will develop.

In this text *chong mai* is not only the director of the circulation of *qi* and the aspect of the circulation which brings nourishment, but also the function which regulates irrigation – carrying fluids and blood throughout the body, even in 'the small and large valleys'. The small and large valleys represent the circulation in the mass of the flesh, from the twelve meridians to the smallest *luo* which irrigate up to the surface of the skin. This is the broadest function of *chong mai*. The *chong mai* seems to be everywhere in the body, from the upper orifices to the bottom of the feet, and from the first centre of the vitality to the most exterior areas of the body, wherever there is circulation of the elements of life, blood and essences.

These classical presentations of pathways are really quite symbolic or emblematic, and the function of *chong mai* is seen everywhere. Great commentators such as Zhang Jiebin said that there is really no place where the *chong mai* does not go. In this text we can see that it gives support to the back, to the area of the kidneys and *ming men*. And *chong mai* has this relationship with the back as well as with the navel and the front of the body. It is able to extend the power of the vitality.

Another important point is to understand the double designation of *chong mai* as it passes over the abdomen; in one text *shao yin* of the foot, the kidney meridian, in another *yang ming* of the foot, the stomach meridian. This is also a way to indicate that *chong mai* makes the connection between pre- and post-heaven, the connection between the first pattern of life and the perpetual renewal of life which follows that pattern.

It is important to consider *chong mai* in the third position, appearing as an emanation from the combination of the two poles of vitality, *yin* and *yang*, represented within the function of the body by *du mai* and *ren mai*. In Chinese, one is written 一, two 二 and three 三. But when the character for three was originally written, one stroke was added, not on the top or bottom but in the middle of the first two. This implies that the third is the result of the communication and exchange between the two.

In Chinese numerology, three is the number for human beings but also for *qi*, because *qi* is the result of the communication between heaven and earth. It is the movement caused by this exchange – heaven is turned towards the earth and earth turned to receive from heaven. Three is the appropriate number for human beings if we take humans as the ultimate expression between heaven and earth, mutually dependent on heaven and earth. The vertical position of human beings was seen as a sign of the ability to communicate with heaven at the time of the Han Dynasty. Laozi chapter 42 says:

'The *dao* produces the one
The one produces the two
The two produces the three
The three produces the 10,000 beings.'

The correct position of human beings is to be between *yin* and *yang*, the harmony for life appearing in this median void. The character for the median void (*chong* 沖) is very close to that of *chong mai*. It is made with the water radical (水), which is used to symbolize all kinds of invisible movements and currents, and the centre (中) which is the space between. From ancient times there has been a correlation between these two characters *chong* (衝) and *chong* (沖). And in modern China the simplified version of *chong* (衝) is *chong* (沖). We can see *chong* as the power of life made through the harmony of the opposites of *yin* and *yang* and all the contrasted powers within a living being made in the pattern of *yin* and *yang* like *xue qi*, blood and *qi*. At this junction and conjunction the power is very broad and can invade everything and create everything.

After three we can of course continue to the four and the five to understand the numerological differentiation step by step, but you can also move directly to the totality, as in Laozi, where the three produce the 10,000. In the *chong mai*, which is the sea of blood, the sea of the *jing luo*, the sea of the meridians, the sea of the five *zang* and six *fu*, *chong mai* is the whole organism, able to go into the smallest and largest valleys throughout the body. This is why sometimes, for example in Suwen chapter 1, it is called the powerful *chong mai*, or the great *chong mai*.

The influence of *chong mai* is seen everywhere in the body, but at the level of the navel, on the kidney meridian, (Ki 16, *huang yu* 肓 俞) there is an injection of vitality. *Huang* (肓) is a kind of membrane, and the source of these membranes is both around the navel and at the centre of the lower abdomen. *Huang* is also found between the diaphragm and the heart. This *huang* is able to envelop all the essential functions and is found wherever something needs to be enveloped and protected; the *huang* line all the hollows where the *qi* and the *zang* and *fu* are found. The connection between *chong mai* and the kidney meridian at the navel, both through the name of this point and also in other texts, shows that these membranes are also the place where the power of *chong mai* can manifest itself.

Chong mai appears to be both the link between, and the manifestation of, a couple, *yin* and *yang*, blood and *qi*, etc. It is also the connection between pre- and post-heaven, stomach and kidneys. It unifies the three levels of the body, the three heaters; it has a relationship with the origin in the centre of the intimate envelope; a relationship with the stomach in the middle heater; and with the pattern of diffusion giving the power to expand and diffuse from the sea of *qi* in the middle of the chest, which is the function of the upper heater.

Or we could see the three parts of the body as the legs, the trunk and the head, and this is the first extraordinary meridian to penetrate the legs and to link the body from below aa well as making the connection with heaven.

Lingshu chapter 33 presents the four seas, and *chong mai* is one of these four seas. It is very unusual to call a meridian a sea. The other seas presented are the stomach, *tan zhong* (膻 中) and the brain. The brain is the sea which receives the finest marrow, and the stomach receives the essences of fluids and grains. As for *tan zhong*, the sea of *qi* in the chest, it unifies the *qi*, and leads the circulation of the *qi* throughout the whole body. But *chong mai* is everywhere and nowhere. It is a sea, but not only that, it is a sea that changes its name. In the first presentation *chong mai* is called the sea of the twelve meridians, and further on in the chapter when the pathological aspect is discussed, *chong mai* is called the sea of blood.

Lingshu chapter 33:

'The stomach is the sea of fluids and grains, its points are above at the street of *qi* (St 30), and below at *san li* (St 36). *Chong mai* is the sea of the twelve meridians, its points are above at *da zhu* (Bl 11), and below at the upper and lower face of the great void (St 37 and 39). *Tan zhong* is the sea of *qi*. Its points are above and below the pillar bone, (Du 14, 15 or Bl 10) and at the front at *ren ying* (St 9). The brain is the sea of marrow, its points are above at the canopy (Du 20) and below at *feng fu* (Du 16).

'In an excess of the sea of blood, one constantly has the sensation of a large body, one is ill at ease (anxious and unhappy) without knowing where the illness is located. If there is insufficiency of the sea of blood one has the sensation of a small body, one is cramped without knowing where the illness is.'

If you consider the special points to treat the four seas, for the stomach both points are on the lower part of the body, for *tan zhong* they are at the neck, for the brain on the skull. But for *chong mai* the points are one at the top of the trunk and two others on the lower limbs. This shows the broad extension of *chong mai*.

As far as the pathology is concerned, it is described as a general feeling, which is everywhere throughout the body. In the case of excess as well as deficiency, one is unable to know exactly where the illness is. If it is really a pathology of *chong mai*, it has repercussions in all the circulation of the meridians and connections, the illness is everywhere. The sensation is to have a large body, as if you are swollen with blood and *qi*, and to be ill at ease as if the skin cannot contain such a large amount of blood and *qi*.

In deficiency it is the opposite, there is a slowing down of the circulation and a diminution in the quantity of blood causing a feeling of shrunkeness. To call *chong mai* 'the sea of the twelve meridians' at the beginning of the chapter and later 'the sea of blood' is a way to show the inter-relationship of blood and *qi*. It represents all the circulation in the meridians, which is nothing other than a good balance between blood and *qi*.

Finally, the sea of blood is sometimes associated with *chong mai*, sometimes with the liver, because the liver also takes part of the function of *chong mai*, which is apparent in gynaecology. The *bao* (胞) or uterus is also called the sea of blood, and this refers not only to the physical uterus, but includes all the functions which allow the uterus to work well – the mechanism for gathering blood in order to allow regular menstruation, and all the regulation of the circulation of blood for a woman.

There is a very strong connection between *chong mai* and the uterus, and if the connection of all this kind of protecting and enveloping in the body, not only the *bao* but also the *huang* (membranes), is also linked to the *chong mai* – for the process of gathering as well as for discharge and emission – we can see why *chong mai* is the sea of blood for menstruation, as well as the sea of blood for the circulation through the meridians and all the network of channels.

Lingshu chapter 65 explains how *chong mai* and *ren mai* give the primitive and structural principles for the circulation of blood:

'When blood and *qi* rise in power, this benefits the skin and the flesh warmed. When only the blood rises in power, a drop by drop infiltration into the layers of the skin provides what is necessary for the growth of the hair.

'Now women in their physiology have an excess of *qi* and an insufficiency of blood, following the frequent loss of blood; *chong mai* and *ren mai* do not make her mouth and lips flourish and because of this she does not have a beard.

'In the case of eunuchs (whether by accident or operation) their ancestral muscle (*zong jin* 宗筋) has gone, their *chong mai* has been attacked, the blood has been dispersed without return, the skin is knotted on the inside; there is no flourishing at the lips and mouth, and this is why the beard does not grow... (With natural eunuchs) there is an insufficiency in their nature (*tian* 天); with them *ren mai* and *chong mai* have not risen in power (*bu sheng* 不盛) and the ancestral muscle (*zong jin* 宗筋) is incomplete (*bu cheng* 不 成); they have *qi*, but not blood; the lips and mouth do not flourish (*bu rong* 不 榮) and because of this the beard does not grow.'

Chong mai and *ren mai* are vital for all the circulation, but they also regulate the distribution of the blood – not only the distribution through the twelve meridians, and through the small and large valleys. They also provide the specific rules within the bodies of the men and women, which of course are not the same. *Ren* and *chong mai* regulate the circulation of blood – for a woman that includes menstruation, for a man it inludes the ability to grow a beard.

In the second part of the text we can see again the important relationship between the *zong jin*, the ancestral muscle or the common point for the muscles, and the *chong mai*. This is another way to show the power of the *chong mai*, because all movement resides in the ancestral muscle, and for a man that includes the ability to sustain an erection and therefore the power of reproduction.

The sea of blood is in this same area, for a men as well as women. That is why when a man is castrated both the muscular forces and the sea of blood are affected, and therefore there is a change in the role of the movement of blood through the *chong mai*. He is unable to grow a beard because the fundamental rulership of the circulation of his blood is changed and altered. It is the same thing with natural eunuchs; here there is a deficiency and an abnormality in the rules of the circulation of blood from the very beginning of life.

Here we can see here the importance of *ren mai* and *chong mai* in all gynaecological and obstetric problems. They are linked in their function to the kidneys, the liver, and maybe the gallbladder for men, and also the heart and spleen is association with the sea of blood.

PATHOLOGY OF CHONG MAI

Nanjing chapter 29:

> 'When *chong mai* gives rise to illnesses the *qi* moves counter (to the normal) current (*ni qi* 逆 氣) and the inside is tense.'

Suwen chapter 60:

> 'When *chong mai* gives rise to illness, the *qi* ascends in a counter-current and the inside is tense.'

Elisabeth Rochat: There is no location for this pathology, just a general indication of a pathology following the function of *chong mai*. *Chong mai* is the sea of all the vital circulation; it is able to direct and stimulate all the circulation because it is everywhere – in the legs as well as the trunk, in the front as well as in the back. This is because it has connections with all the meridians, or connections coming from the meridians. It is the main highway from which all other circulation diverges.

There is a connection with this character *chong* (衝) with

another character *tong* (通) meaning free circulation. If the *chong mai* is unable to ensure free circulation and good communication, if it is unable to ensure a good direction for the *qi*, with the right proportion of *qi*, blood and essences, then that is a 'counter-current'. When the text says that the 'inside is tense' it suggests a kind of contraction within the organism, perhaps due to a weakness and diminution of blood and *yin* which is then unable to irrigate the muscles. This pathology is similar to the pathology of the sea of blood in Lingshu chapter 33, with no specific location and no specific symptoms. The *chong mai* is implicated wherever there is a problem with the circulation – not just involving one or two meridians, but more general. If there is a lack of nourishment by the *yin* everywhere in the body, that can be seen as a pathology of *chong mai*.

Normally and practically speaking, disturbances of *chong mai* are often linked to an irregularity in the distribution of blood, especially for women. This is a practical application of the most general pathological indication of *chong mai*. This pathology is related to the *qi*, but also to all kinds of fluids circulating with the *qi*. The *jin mai* (筋 脈) is a system of distribution within the small and large valleys of the flesh and the muscles. It is the circulation of blood and *qi* and essences which are necessary for movement and the nourishment of the muscles. If there is a kind of contraction in the interior of the body, this may be a general pathology affecting the *jin mai*, which refers to the regular movement, nourishment and irrigation of the muscles. Here we can see a connection with the liver and gallbladder, and also the spleen and stomach.

If the counter-current of *qi* occurs in the chest at the level of the sea of *qi*, it would cause pain, possibly in the heart. And that is why some pains in the heart are related to *chong mai*. There may also be pain and discomfort in the thorax with a feeling of being stifled, and respiratory disturbance, especially shortness of breath. Many different kinds of symptoms related to problems with the circulation of blood and *qi* throughout the trunk may come under the authority of *chong mai* if there is a very general pattern of disorder.

Question: Is it possible to say a little about when you would decide to treat *ren mai* or *chong mai* in gynaecological problems, rather than say the spleen or the liver?

Elisabeth Rochat: It is up to each practitioner to have their own vision of the human life and the body. In this vision the eight extraordinary meridians are just the first structure, but we have to deal with the present condition of the person in front of us and we can make a diagnosis only in terms of ordinary meridians and *zang* and *fu*. For instance through the kidneys, and the interplay between the kidneys and stomach, it is possible to treat even the deep and structural root of the person. But you can also enlarge that and have a different approach.

When more than one or two *zang* or meridians are involved, just think about the principles behind these two *zang* or *fu* or meridians. When it seems that a specific function is involved, for example that it is something to do with the blood, or something to do with the general organization of the circulation of *qi*, or something to do with a general weakness of *yin*, or a general weakness of *yang*, you can treat each of the *zang* and *fu* and meridians concerned, or you can see it in terms of the extraordinary meridians, which are like the common basis of all the meridians. And as far as treatment is concerned, I think that there is no difference, because whether the diagnosis is made with the extraordinary meridians, or the *zang* and *fu* and meridians, the points may be the same. Often with a *zang* and *fu* diagnosis you may choose to use points which are also points for the extraordinary meridians. You can also have the opposite approach, beginning your reasoning with the extraordinary meridians and adding other points for the complete treatment.

There are special techniques taught in schools on the extraordinary meridians, which are very well documented, for example, in the book 'The Extraordinary Vessels' by Matsumoto and Birch (Paradigm Publications). This is a very good clinical study of all the Japanese techniques using the extraordinary meridians.

For specific problems, for example with menstruation, there may be a relationship with one of the five *zang*, but generally speaking you can also use *ren* and *chong mai*. It is of course possible to make a more specific connection between *chong mai* and the spleen and liver for these kinds of problems, or with *ren mai* and the liver, spleen and kidney meridians, too. It is important to see that *ren mai* is more concerned with the *yin* and the blood itself, with the production and the conservation of the blood, whereas *chong mai* is rather more concerned with the power of the blood and the correct working of the physiological function through the movement of the blood. But at that level the answer is always in your practice.

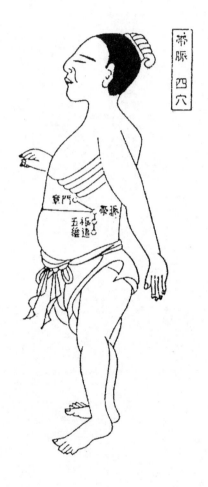

Dai mai from the Neiwaigong tushuo

DAI MAI 帶 脈

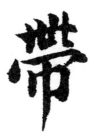

Elisabeth Rochat: Dai mai (帶 脈) has the meaning of a belt and the etymology is quite simple. The character *dai* (帶) depicts a garment held together by a belt or girdle. But it is not simply a belt, like a ribbon or a strap, because there is also the possibility of attaching something, to have something hanging from the belt. The ancient Chinese custom was to have jade, jewellery, tablets and other things hanging from the belt. According to Wieger, the etymology represents a girdle with three trinkets hanging from it.

But this character has other meanings which are also related to the function of *dai mai*. It can be any kind of band which assures the continuity of something, like a current of water or a chain of several mountains. Another series of meanings is to be able to lead, to guide or to drive something, and these meanings are derived from the ability to attach and to hold firmly. It also means 'to conduct', and if you add the character *dao* (道), the way or the route, it gives the expression to guide on a route, or in shipping it is the pilot ship which guides larger ships into the port.

The character can also express the idea of connections and relationships – being close together and acting for the same purpose. If we add the radical for vegetation (蔕) the meaning is the stalk or stem of a flower, the part of the flower that is close to the roots, close to the base or foundation and not just something added. It is central and fundamental to the power of guidance and of holding things firmly and conducting them well.

Claude Larre: To confirm what Elisabeth has said, I would refer you to lesson 16 A in Wieger, where a garment is described as a robe dragging on the ground. But when the character *dai* is used, the cloth is well arranged, there is no dragging or moving around. So the character has the idea of arrangement and control: to keep carefully and in the correct place.

Elisabeth Rochat: This character *dai* (帶) can also have the meaning of abnormal discharges, especially vaginal discharge in women.

If we look at the classical commentators, they give us the idea of a belt, but a belt which extends and binds. And this is compared to the way in which a bundle of sticks is bound together, firmly, where not one stick is able to move. *Dai mai* is given this name because its function is to bind together and at the same time to unify all the *mai*. This is the impression of Li Shizhen, who wrote a complete treatise on the extraordinary meridians in the second part of the 16th century.

Other commentators have said that as well as this ability to hold all the *mai* together it also has the role of harmonizing and regulating them, and we will see that from the texts of the Neijing and Nanjing.

Finally, there is another character which is very important in Chinese pathology – *zhi* (滯), which means blockage, and is one of the characters most frequently used for pathological blockage. It is made with the character *dai* and the radical for water; the original meaning is ice. This suggests that the action of this belt is able to condense water right up to the point of freezing – the water being condensed more and more until it solidifies. This kind of blockage is caused by constraint, so the belt must be tight enough, but not too constricting.

Dai mai is not so much a line on the surface, but the entire cross-section of the body at this level. It is an important way to harmonize and regulate all the pathways of vital circulation, and all the meridians passing the influential area of *dai mai*. It is like a horizontal band, with the function of regulating all this movement, not only binding together, but exerting a very well balanced pressure, and thus regulating the flow up and down all the meridians.

The character *zhi* (滯) suggests the kind of blockage where the *dai mai* is constricted and *dai* (帶) suggests general discharges, where the *dai mai* is too relaxed.

THE PATHWAY OF DAI MAI

Nanjing chapter 28:

> '*Dai mai* arises from the last ribs; it turns once around the body.'

This trajectory of *dai mai* is like a belt, sloping forwards, and taking under its authority the area of the origin and the inner power – which we have seen with the joint origin of *du mai*, *ren mai* and *chong mai*. Of course, women's reproductive organs are at this level, which is one of the explanations of the importance of *dai mai* in the correct function of the uterus, and the balance of fluids, blood and the possibility of dampness in the lower heater, especially for women. The connection with the area of *ming men* (命 門) and the special *yu* point of the kidneys (*shen shu* 腎 俞 Bl 23) is found in Lingshu chapter 11 in the description of the detached pathway of the kidney meridian (*jing bie* 經 別):

> 'The correct (*zheng* 正) of the *shao yin* of the foot (ie. the principal pathway of the kidney meridian) reaches the back of the knee and detaches (*bie* 別); it (the detached part) goes to the *tai yang* to which it unites (*he* 合). It rises and reaches the height of the 14th vertebra; it leaves and takes a dependent (*shu* 屬) relation with *dai mai*. The pathway goes off directly to connect with the root of the tongue. Again it detaches at the nape of the neck, and reunites with the *tai yang*, this is the first reunion (or junction, *he* 合).'

These reunions (or junctions, *he* 合) are the six reunions (*liu he* 六合) that the twelve meridians have through their *bie* (別), separate or divergent pathways. What is important here is that the *bie* of the kidney meridian has a special relationship with the *dai mai*. It is a relationship of dependency (*shu* 屬) which indicates that the quality of *qi* is the same. For example the kidney meridian has a *shu* relationship with the viscera of the kidneys, and this suggests a community of *qi* which belongs to the same family.

Another important thing is that the level of this conjunction is the 14th vertebra, which is the area of *ming men* (命 門 Du 4) and *shen yu* (腎 俞 Bl 23). So *dai mai* is firmly anchored at *ming men* and connected with the power of the kidneys; and though the *jing bie*, which is the deep and inner pathway, there is a relationship with the kidneys and with the kidney and bladder meridians. This connection with the kidneys and *ming men* gives *dai mai* its relationship with the origin, and the origin as it expresses itself on the back, in the area of *yang*, of *du mai* and of the kidneys.

The presentation of the pathway in later texts give a more usual description, for example in Li Shizhen:

'*Dai mai* surges from the point *zhang men* (章 門 Liv 13) on the *jue yin* of the foot, by the lower ribs. Together with the *shao yang* of the foot it runs along the point *dai mai* (帶 脈 Gb 26). It makes a complete circuit of the body, like a belt which is tied together. It meets the *shao yang* of the foot again at *wu shu* (五 樞 Gb 27) and *wei dao* (維 道 Gb 28). Altogether eight points.'

POINTS OF DAI MAI

Liver 13 *zhang men* 章門

The first point mentioned here is Liver 13 *zhang men* (章門). This point has two particular attributes: one is to be the meeting (*hui* 合) point of the five *zang*, and the other to be the *mu* point for the spleen. So it has an action on the five deep *yin* viscera and also it is the *mu* point of the spleen. As the spleen is the centre of the five *zang* it is quite natural that we should find this point for both. The very close connection between *dai mai* and the spleen can also be seen in the control of fluids and their circulation in the middle and lower heaters.

Gallbladder 26 *dai mai* 帶脈

This point is at the level of the umbilicus and with the name *dai mai* the meaning of this point gives the same idea of binding and connecting all the *mai*.

Gallbladder 27 *wu shu* 五樞

Wu shu is translated as five pivots. Five is a totality, but always a totality around a centre. *Dai mai* is related to the middle heater and all the inner forces of life – through the five *zang* and *ming men* and the kidneys. It expresses this power as a belt holding all the *mai*, like a central axis, for a totality of rotation and circulation. It enables circulation between the upper and lower parts of the body as well as for the *qi* coming from the five *zang*. The number five suggests that this activity is all well regulated and harmonized because there is a centre. And of course this point is on the gallbladder meridian, and we must not forget that *shao yang* is the pivot.

Anatomically speaking this is an area where the musculature is quite interesting; it is the meeting of the internal and external oblique muscles. Gallbladder 27 is nearly at the same height as *guan yuan* (關 元) Ren 4, and on the stomach meridian as *shui dao* (水 道) St 28. There is a suggestion of the ability to command movement in all directions.

Claude Larre: The name *shu* (樞) implies a verticality given by the tree radical on the left of the character, which gives the impression of revolving parts, a bit like a revolving door.

Gallbladder 28 *wei dao* 維 道

Elisabeth Rochat: Dao (道) is the way, and *wei* (維) is the same character used for *yin* and *yang wei mai*, the power to attach, to moor something. Another name for this point is *wai shu* (外 樞), the external pivot, or the pivot turned towards the exterior. *Wei dao* suggests the correct conduction, well maintained as if kept in a net, and attached as if with a mooring. It suggests the correct maintenance and protection of all the pathways of the *yin* and *yang mai* throughout the body; a combining of all routes and pathways.

This point is very close to the insertion point of the sartorius muscle, and the sartorius has a connection with the knee, which may explain some of the pathology of *dai mai* in connection with the lower limbs. This interplay of *dai mai* with the muscles would make a very interesting study.

These three points of the gallbladder meridian give the impression of holding something, and not just holding but ensuring good conduction and free circulation – in a very supervised kind of freedom.

Li Shizhen:

'Yangshi says: *dai mai* takes all the *mai* under its command by linking them; it ensures that there is no erratic circulation, like a man who ties together a belt which hangs at the front. Hence its name.'

There is a relationship in the description of *dai mai* with *ming men* and the kidneys, and through the kidneys and *ming men* to the whole area of the origin of the *du mai*. There is also a relationship with the liver and gallbladder, which are the pivot between *yin* and *yang*, and the *shao yang* in particular, which is the pivot between the *biao* and the *li*, the interior and the exterior. The liver and gallbladder meridians are the pivot because they are on the side of the body and the *dai mai* is also like a pivot but at the centre, ensuring regular circulation between the lower and upper parts of the body.

Some commentators emphasize the relationship with the spleen, especially in the pathology of *dai mai* which is related to vaginal discharges. *Chong mai* is the connection between the kidneys and original *qi* and the stomach, the middle heater and post-heaven – or the renewal of life from the exterior in the form of food and air which is assimilated into the body. *Dai mai* has a similar role, making a link between the kidneys and the spleen, especially in relation to the control of fluids, which we will see in the pathology.

The power of *dai mai* comes from the strength in the area of the back that is related to the kidneys, and from its expression through the liver and gallbladder, which are the physical upsurge of life. The ability of *dai mai* to hold and to suspend is also very close to one of the functions of the spleen. We will see with the pathology of *dai mai* that the ability of the circulation to go down to the extremity of the limbs is to do with having the right kind of tension; not too relaxed and not too tight. This will also be seen in the relationship between *dai mai* and the ancestral muscle.

PATHOLOGY OF DAI MAI

Elisabeth Rochat: All the pathologies of *dai mai* are related to the functions that we have already seen. Generally there may be congestion which hampers circulation in the abdomen. There can also be weakness in the lumbar area, with, as it says in the Nanjing, 'the feeling of sitting in water'. The pathology of *dai mai* given in the Neijing and Nanjing often concerns gynaecology, particularly vaginal discharge, which is differentiated into two categories, red or white: with or without blood, with heat or with cold. Remember that through the link with the spleen and kidneys there is this control of fluids, water and dampness.

For women, *dai mai* also controls the uterus, *bao* (胞), and the function of the uterus as the sea of blood; it organizes the circulation and distribution of blood in a woman's body, and regulates the menstrual flow. We have seen this with *chong mai* and the liver. If there is weakness in the meridians at that level and the pathways are too loose, there may be discharge. As all the pathways of the meridians have a relationship with *dai mai*, if *dai mai* is not able to ensure circulation it is very easy for dampness, cold or heat to stagnate around the lumbar area and the belly.

There can also be symptoms in the muscles related to *dai mai*, for example pain around the navel radiating to the lumbar area and the spine. There may also be violent pain in the sides of the back. Sometimes there can be menstrual disturbance.

If the *dai mai* is affected by cold, there is a tightening and all the meridians will have problems in their circulation because of this constriction. If there is heat, there can be a scattering and disorder in the meridians. We must not forget that if *dai mai* has its point of anchorage at Liver 13, this also suggests a relationship to the diaphragm.

Through its relationship with the inner part of the belly, *dai mai* is also related to the common origin of *du mai, ren mai* and *chong mai* which is the *bao zhong* (胞 中) or intimate envelope. Many commentators stress the influence of *dai mai* in making the complete interconnection between the first four extraordinary meridians in this area of the origin.

Nanjing difficulty 29:

> 'When *dai mai* gives rise to illnesses, the abdomen is congested, the lumbar area is like flowing water, and one feels as if one is sitting in water.'

This kind of congestion in the abdomen is due to the loosening of *dai mai* which is unable to transport and transform fluids and dampness. This causes swelling and congestion due to accumulated fluids, and is why we have this expression of water flowing in the lumbar area. It is a kind of congestion with stagnation and pervading cold. These symptoms also show a weakness of the kidneys, as the kidneys are unable to master water and cold, and also weakness of the spleen because the spleen is unable to transform dampness and fluids and assimilate them into the organism.

The expression 'to be seated in water' is a way to express this feeling of cold and lack of strength in the lumbar area. If you sit in cold water for a long time you become unable to move easily, especially to move the lower limbs, and there is a real lack of strength. All movements are hard, painful and slow.

The commentators give many symptoms related to this

particular pathology: all kinds of gynaecological discharges from damp, and in men certain *shan* (疝) syndromes, including swelling and congestion in the lower abdomen, and especially those linked to the pathology of the liver and gallbladder with swellings and numbness. There may, for example, be cold in the liver meridian because *dai mai* is unable to regulate the circulation in this area. As usual with extraordinary meridian symptoms, they are very general. If we look at the symptoms linked with the liver meridian in the Lingshu there is a very precise description of certain *shan* syndromes, but this is not the case with the extraordinary meridian pathologies. The symptoms affect the circulation in the whole area of the lower abdomen.

Claude Larre: Vague and general symptoms are normal in the pathology of the extraordinary meridians because they are at the level of life where precise distinction has not yet taken place. The body itself is not distinct, it is still under the influence of the primitive state of the embryo, slowly developing more precise functions. Even in the adult, there is always a link with this less defined condition, which is the reason for the more vague description in the pathology.

Elisabeth Rochat: We can also see that certain schools of commentators in China said that if the kidneys are cold, and if there is a weakness coming from the origin, a deficiency of the *yang* of the kidneys and *ming men*, there will be weakness in the strength of the liver and gallbladder, and this is called 'a decreasing of the *qi* of the *yang* coming from the depths of the *yin*'. The *yang* of the liver and the gallbladder are rooted in the kidney *yin*, with consequences to circulation in the lower heater and the control of the lower orifices. That is also a way to indicate the relationship of *dai mai* with the liver and gallbladder meridians. The points of the *dai mai* are points on these meridians.

The commentator Zhangjing said that this kind of *dai mai* pathology could also appear after a long illness, causing the same decrease of *yang* at that level. In this case one should tonify with herbs and use moxa on Liver 13 (*zhang men* 章 門) which would affect the liver and the spleen, and strengthen the *yin* of the five *zang* in order to invigorate the *yang* of the *yin*.

Suwen chapter 44:

'*Yin* and *yang* meet together at the ancestral muscle (*zong jin* 宗 筋); they meet at the street of *qi* (*qi jie* 氣 街 St 30) and the *yang ming* is the most important. All this maintains a relation of dependence (*shu* 屬) with the *dai mai* and a relation of connection (*luo* 絡) with the *du mai*.

'When *yang ming* is empty, the ancestral muscle is relaxed (*zong* 縱) the *dai mai* no longer guides (*yin* 引) and for this reason, the lower limbs are impotent (*wei* 痿) and can no longer function.'

This *wei* (痿) pathology originates from within the body, and the weakness is caused by a lack of irrigation, moistening and movement in the muscles. That is why there is this kind of impotence. It begins at the feet and there may be problems with the knees, or flaccidity and numbness or paralysis in the muscles of the legs. Many kinds of symptoms are possible, this is just the general pattern.

One meaning of *wei* (瘘) is sexual impotence, and this is when the ancestral muscle is attacked at the perineum; the mechanism is exactly the same.

Impotence in the lower limbs is due to the *dai mai* and here the weakness of *dai mai* is caused by weakness of the stomach and of post-heaven *qi*. The strength of *dai mai* is comes from the origin, from the original *qi*, but in order to maintain and rebuild this strength it must be nourished through the activity of the spleen and stomach. If the stomach is unable to provide essences and fluids and sufficient irrigation, the releasing of *qi* will also gradually diminish, and the circulation in the four limbs will be unable to nourish and moisten the muscles.

As well as being in charge of holding, *dai mai* is also in charge of controlling circulation, especially in the lower limbs. It conducts the *qi* of the whole organism in the right direction and to the right place. This character *yin* (引), Weiger lesson 87 A, is made with a bow, but it also contains the image of a rope with the correct tension. With an extra stroke it means to draw the string of a bow, and by extension, to attract, to lead, to induce, to seduce. It is a good character for the *dai mai*, to induce and to conduct. The image is the same as that of the expression *dao yin* (導 引).

As always, this function or ability has two sides. For example, the kidneys control water, essences and *yin* in the body, but they are also responsible for the overflow of fluids. It is the same with the *dai mai*. It ensures this binding, but it must be with a kind of relaxation. If it is too relaxed there is erratic circulation, congestion and knotting. If it is too tight there will be other kinds of blockage and congestion. It must be able to keep a good balance between what goes up and what goes down. It must be able to control the circulation of fluids and dampness, not allowing it to overflow, for example as vaginal discharge or swellings in the genitals. But it is also in charge of making this circulation function in the lower limbs.

Let us look at some of the other classical indications found in Li Shizhen:

'*Dai mai* (Gb 26) masters all the symptoms mentioned in Nanjing 29. A loosening in the lumbar area and the belly with the feeling of cooling as if seated in cold water.

'For women, the lower belly is painful with cramping and contractions, with the feeling of wanting to defecate. Disturbances in menstruation and red or white vaginal discharge. Needle 6 fen and moxa 7 times.'

Liver 13 (*zhang men* 章 門) is given in other texts for these symptoms, again with the use of moxa. Liver 13 is also given for different kinds of *shan* syndrome, for example painful swelling in the testicles, particularly in young boys.

DAI XIA 帶下

Elisabeth Rochat: An important pathology of the *dai mai* is *dai xia*. Dai (帶) is the *dai* of *dai mai*, *xia* (下) is to go down, suggesting that at the level of the *dai mai*, something is going down.

Li Shizhen:

'In women, discharges follow *dai mai* to descend. Hence the name *dai xia* (abnormal discharges in women). It is mentioned that a woman can suffer from red discharges or white discharges. Some moxa *qi hai* (氣海 Ren 6) and if it is not sufficient the following day they moxa the point *dai mai* (帶脈 Gb 26).'

Liu Zonghou says:

'Women's discharges, *dai xia*, are fundamentally an emptiness of *yin* and an exhaustion of *yang* (*yin xu yang jie* 陰虛陽竭). The nutritive *qi* (*ying qi* 營氣) does not rise, the meridians are congealed and circulate poorly; the defensive *qi* (*wei qi* 衛氣) collapses below; the *jing qi* (精氣) accumulates and becomes blocked in the lower heater, in the area of the extraordinary meridians, *qi mai* (奇脈); this leads to accumulation and fermentation which causes illness in the *dai mai*. Hence the name *dai xia*.

'When it is white it is related to the *qi*, when it is red it is related to the blood.

'The causes are especially from eating and drinking too much, from exhaustion or from excessive sexual activity. It can also be that dampness and phlegm pour out and flow into the lower heater; the *yin* of the liver and kidneys is uncontrolled and dampness prevails.

'In other cases one is subject to movements of fear and fright; wood overrides the earth and unclear fluids flow out below. Or worries and preoccupations are endless, and set off muscular impotence (*jin wei* 筋痿), this causes the illnesses of the second *yang* to be released to the heart and the spleen.

'Or there is an excess of dampness and heat which forces the belt (*dai* 帶) in the lower abdomen to give way. Or the lower origin is empty and cold, the palace of the child (the womb) is damp and without control...'

This cause of vaginal discharges due to worries and preoccupations is similar to that in Suwen chapter 44:

'When obsessive thought holds sway indefinitely and one does not obtain what one aspires to, when the intention (*yi* 意) flows out uncontrollably to the exterior and one spends one's intensity in the bedroom [excessive sexual activity], the ancestral muscle (*zong jin* 宗筋) becomes completely spent. This causes muscular impotence (*jin wei* 筋痿) to the point that there is uncontrollable leaking of the white substance [vaginal discharges or spermatorrhoea].'

The cause of this situation is internal obstruction due to worries and preoccupations, or obsessive thinking and the fire of desire – possibly a kind of sexual obsession, or the desire of something which cannot be obtained. This inner agitation due to unsatisfied desire leads to loss of blood and fluids. This causes a decline of *yin* and essences, and a lack of moistening and nourishing of the muscles, especially the ancestral muscle.

The text then presents various kinds of muscular impotence throughout the body, especially in the lower limbs, and a kind of loosening in the lower abdomen which leads to these white discharges. These patterns have a relationship with *dai mai*, but also with *ren mai* and *chong mai* in their control over the lower abdomen and especially with gynaecology. The liver, the spleen and the kidneys are also involved.

Dai xia is caused by blockage due to dampness which causes a kind of inner fermentation. The problem occurs in the *bao*, the intimate envelope or uterus. At the same time there is an emptiness of the spleen which is unable to transform dampness, and the *dai mai* loses its power to conduct and to hold.

Dai xia caused by desire and obsessive thinking can also lead to an attack on the spleen, causing blockage at the level of the liver or the heart by dampness and heat. Suppressed anger can also cause this kind of blockage with an attack from the liver to the spleen. And there may also be difficulties after delivery.

SUMMARY OF DAI MAI

Elisabeth Rochat: So, what is this new stage reached with *dai mai*? It is not simply a circle around the body, but an expression of the volume of the whole body. *Du mai* governs the back, *ren mai* the front; *chong mai* is in the centre. But this gives just two dimensions; *dai mai* gives us the volume – it is like inflating a balloon. The *dai mai* comes from within, and gives an expansion of volume, while at the same time giving a limit to this expansion. From its position at the centre of the body, it holds all circulation and inter-connections in place. This is why the *dai mai* is associated with the 'six junctions'. But remember that the six junctions are the four directions plus height and depth. Here the plan is expanded into a living area, which is also found in the the reunions of the twelve meridians through the *jing bie* (經別); to build and to limit the area of life – to give volume but also to contain and close. So in *dai mai* there is always the function of maintaining the relationship between the height and the depths.

Even though *dai mai* has this horizontal position, it is not a *luo*. Because although the *luo* (絡) are generally transversal and horizontal and the meridians are vertical, *dai mai* is definitely a *jing* (經), a meridian, because it provides a norm for the circulation. It provides a pattern for the regulation and good balance of all the circulation within the body. We will see the *luo* function with the *qiao mai*.

As far as *du mai, ren mai, chong mai* and *dai mai* are concerned, there is no anchorage in the limbs. *Chong mai* descends to the bottom of the foot but it begins at the centre. Only the *qiao mai* and *wei mai* have their beginning and anchoring in the lower limbs. But the pathologies of the extraordinary meridians have symptoms of the whole body. The mastery of the *du mai* is over all the *yang* meridians and all the *yang* functions in the body, and the mastery of the *ren mai* is over all the *yin* functions throughout the body. The pathology of the *dai mai* concerns the lower limbs, the deficiency of the function of *dai mai* leading to a relaxation of the muscles in the thighs and legs.

Claude Larre: The separation of the eight extraordinary meridians falls quite naturally into four and four. The *dai mai* closes the first series. Being the fourth, the only possible position is to encircle the previous three like a girdle. It has to be at that horizontal level to complete the geometrical construction, because the body is spherical, especially if we are talking about the embryo or the newly born child where the limbs are not yet developed. The power of life is greater at its beginning than at its end, so what has been the initiating force for life will continue after the other energetic pathways are developed.

Dai mai is the ability to make communication between what is above and what is below, but this excludes the limbs. The limbs are more defined with *yin* and *yang qiao mai*. When there are three *mai*, and even when there are four, we are inclined to use numerology to define what comes first, and what comes next, and then to see what develops between them. The four is an extension of what is seen at level of three, and the three is what surges from the fact that between the two a third possibility is welcomed.

But this numerology is only a pattern to help us understand that life is a unity, because Chinese numerology starts from one and always returns to one; for example one is one but two is a couple which is the unity of the two parts joining again. If the two as a couple has to find a way to keep the unity of the two, the third coming between the one and the two, makes three, but the three is seen as a kind of family of life, so life is unique even if it is presented as the number three. And whatever is true for the individual is true for the community of all beings. The community of beings is seen on the earth, earth contains and sustains them, and this is the extension to the number four.

We can go on to five which is the organization of power, the relationship between three and three which is six, and the emerging of life which is the surging between three and three, which is seven, in the same way that three was surging between two. Seven may be extended to eight, and again there is a view of life in the completeness of the eight, in the same way that the three extended to the four directions. If we want to replenish all that is possible with the eight then we come to nine and it is finished. The most essential numerology is always from one to nine. We can start again with ten to have more complexity but we always have to refer back to the first nine.

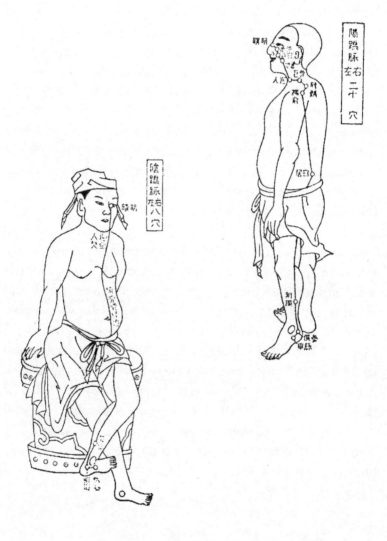

Yin and yang qiao mai

QIAO MAI 蹻 脈

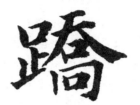

Elisabeth Rochat: The radical of *qiao* (蹻) is the character for foot (足); this indicates the importance of the *qiao mai* for the lower limbs. They begin at the feet. This radical (*zu* 足) is the character that is used to describe the six meridians of the legs. The right part of the character is the phonetic (*qiao* 喬) and describes a kind of pavilion; the meaning will change according to the radical. Combined with the radical 'woman' (嬌) it means something very delicate, fragile and refined; with the radical 'horse' (驕) it is an untamed wild creature, or someone who is arrogant, violent and full of fire. There is both a contrast and a similarity between the two meanings of this character – it suggests the ability to rise up very fiercely but it is also something delicate – which may suggest that if you are at the top you are in the most delicate position.

Claude Larre: I would suggest that this ambivalence is in our minds but not in the reality of life. Because if something is really high, this suggests that it is moving, and when it is moving it is full of grace and refinement, like bamboo in the wind. But if the movement is of someone highly placed in society, their position may create envy in others. If people have high ideals, there will often be envy and animosity around them. The nobility of an animal is seen in its head and hair, and in classical Chinese thought there is a connection between the horse and the heavenly understanding of life. If this character is attributed to a horse, it is quite appropriate, but if it is attributed to a person, then the meaning becomes that of arrogance, haughtiness, etc.

It is important not to immediately attach a particular word to the translation of this character but to return to the lively impression that we have when we think of a horse, or a Tang dynasty court dancer, and from that to understand the meaning according to what we see in life. That is the only way to understand the meaning, which depends upon the radical and the context. If women wear high heeled shoes and their hair on top of their head they are often the envy of other women and men may easily be seduced!

Elisabeth Rochat: So the meaning of this character *qiao* (蹻) with the foot radical is to stand, but to stand in a dynamic way; it is the ability to be erect and to attract energy from the earth up to the top of the body. It can also mean to stand on tiptoes – which is to be higher, but also less stable. There may be some danger with this fierce upward impulse, but it is necessary for both the strength and 'springing up' of life.

Qiao also means agility. If you can lift up your feet and move your legs well, you are able to run, and to run fast. But the meaning of *qiao* is not only to be agile and fast, it is also to be fierce. It can also mean to be robust with a kind of martial temperament, to act with a certain amount of arrogance and pride.

Generally, the explanation for the meaning of *qiao mai* given by classical commentators is rapid: to be able to run rapidly or to hasten. The commentators of the Nanjing say that the ability to run and walk with agility suggests that the *qiao mai* provide the mechanism for walking; it is the ability to move with ease and speed, because the rising up movement of the *qiao mai* gives a feeling of lightness.

Sometimes *qiao* is written another way (蹺). The etymological meaning here is in Wieger lesson 81 C. The top of the phonetic is the earth character (土) repeated three times, which suggests earth heaped up, and with the bottom part, meaning high, the complete explanation is a knoll or a mound. This is the name of the very famous Emperor Yao. It is interesting to see that this character gives the same idea of height, but without the suggestion of being on tiptoes and in danger of over-balancing. This alternative character has the meaning of something very well rooted, very firm and solid, and this is certainly another meaning of the *qiao mai*, to be firmly rooted in the earth – in order to pile up and build the movement of the body.

Claude Larre: If we think of the roots of plants and the ability of plants to take sustenance from their roots, we can see that in order to extend upwards you have to rely on something. In the Chinese view you can never look at the beauty of the expression of life without also looking at the foundations.

Elisabeth Rochat: To see the difference between the two characters we can add the radical for a woman to this second character (嬈), where the meaning is of something graceful, but without the sense of delicacy. With the horse (*xiao* 驍) it is a finely bred horse, fierce or untamed. With the sun (*xiao* 曉) it means to become clear, to gain understanding and knowledge: the light of knowledge. With the radical for a human being (僥) it is to be a happy, fortunate person.

Claude Larre: If you are studying Chinese, it is interesting to look through the tables of radicals and to see for example which words include the radical for the horse. You will find allusions to the colour and the speed of the horse, but also many kinds of behaviour, for example to be frightened or to be haughty. Because the horse is given many of the attributes of heaven, it is often used to describe psychological traits. With the wood radical (橋) it has the meaning of a bridge, especially a very high bridge which allows boats to pass underneath. We see this character in many names of bridges; in Tokyo, for example, it is in the name Nihonbashii.

PATHWAYS OF YIN AND YANG QIAO MAI

Elisabeth Rochat: These two meridians flow from the heels to the top of the head, building something up from the base to the summit. The pathway is given in Nanjing difficulty 28:

'*Yang qiao mai* arises from the middle of the heel; it passes over the external malleolus and penetrates *feng chi* (風 池 Gb 20).

'*Yin qiao mai* also arises from the middle of the heel; it passes over the internal malleolus and rises; it reaches the pharynx; it crosses then joins the *chong mai*.'

The beginning is the same for the *yin* and *yang qiao mai*. Both arise from the heel (*gen* 跟). This character is made with the radical for the foot (足) and if you replace this with the wood radical it is the character for root (*gen* 根). When it is written like this (跟) the character for heel is simply a description of the way that a human being is rooted in the earth and is able to keep contact with the earth through the heels.

In Zhuangzi there is a description of breathing through the heels. This is a method to take breath not only from heaven but also to take the influences of the earth and make them rise up through the body. In this case the heel is designated with another character (*zhong* 踵) which has the same foot radical (*zu* 足) but with a different phonetic. It gives the idea of a root drawing some kind of sap from the depths of the earth and making it rise up through the trunk to the branches. In this character there is again the idea of a piling up, a heaping up, to make something solid and firm. So the heel contains the same double idea: to be firm and solid, through a kind of piling up, and through this accumulation to have an ascending movement.

Claude Larre: Elisabeth was referring to the character for heel as a phonetic, but it is also a radical. The meaning of a character depends on both the phonetic and the radical, and sometimes the phonetic is even more important than the radical to ascertain the meaning. If we want to understand what this character *gen* (跟) means we have to study the radical. This is given in Wieger lesson 26 L. This character *gen* (跟) is also the name of the trigram for mountain, which can be interpreted either as a physical mountain or as a representation of an ascending movement. Since there are eight trigrams, they encompass all types of movement within the universe.

As Elisabeth said, it is not only the *yang* that is rising with these two meridians but also the *yin*, and it is not only the rising movement that is suggested by the characters, but also the place that enables that rising up movement. It is important to take the *yin* and *yang* as a double reference to something which cannot be named, and here we must return to the unknown source from which life emerges. We are not able to understand or describe the unknown, but at least we are able to place things where they are, and from that invisible place we may make further analogies to the *yin* and *yang* aspect: the *yin* and *yang* aspects of the movement of life, and the transformation of the *yin* and *yang* by the merging in the third position. So when considering the beginnings of the *yin* and the *yang* movements, we must also consider what is behind that in order to be true to life. Etymology does not always give the meaning as such, but just a suggestion of the meaning; it is more a description of a picture of the manifestation.

Elisabeth Rochat: *Yang* and *yin qiao mai* begin at the same place: at the heel, not at the malleolus. The centre of the heel corresponds to the function of *qiao*; it is not simply at the heel, but specifically at the centre of the heel. In Unschuld's translation of the Nanjing he just says in the heel, which is correct, but this character *zhong* (中) is usually used to stress that the *qiao mai* remain in the centre, and remain connected with the central organization of the vitality.

The *yang qiao mai* passes over the external malleolus and penetrates *feng chi* (風 池 Gb 20). The external malleolus gives an opposition with the *yin qiao*. They have a common origin, and then the external malleolus is mentioned for the *yang*, the internal malleolus for the *yin*. In this kind of text that differentiation is important because all the relationships between the *qiao mai* are also relationships between the inner and the outer. At the origin in the heel there is communication between the *yin* and *yang*, internal and external. This describes the way that the *yin* and *yang qiao* form a unity within a system, and within the system they are responsible for balance – the equilibrium between *yin* and *yang*, of interior and exterior and so on. We will see that throughout all the other texts, and it is one of the main differences with the *yin* and *yang wei mai* which have more separate systems. For the *qiao mai* it is always a question of balance and exchange between the *yin* and the *yang* but within the one complete system. Their common origin is just an example of that.

In this text, no other points are mentioned but Gallbladder 20, which is the last point of the *yang qiao mai*, and a connection with the nape of the neck – although we know that the *qiao mai* also pass over the head and influence the brain.

In Nanjing 28, the trajectory of *du mai* was said to rise up to *feng fu*, (風 府 Du 16), where *du mai* penetrates and takes a belonging relationship (*shu* 屬) to the brain. So here there is a similarity between *du mai* and *yang qiao mai*, and of course in later texts, they form a couple, as does *yin qiao mai* with *ren mai*. In Lingshu 21 we will see that both *qiao mai* penetrate the brain. The link with *feng chi* (風 池 Gb 20), is probably related to the rapidity of the *qiao*. This kind of pond (*chi* 池) is a natural gathering place for something, a place which stores but also attracts the wind. And there is also a link with the gallbladder meridian, the *shao yang*, which has this same quality of *qi* – to be brave, fierce and rapid.

The *yin qiao mai* rises from the internal malleolus, and it is important to understand that the *yin qiao mai* also has this great power and ability to rise, which is not always the case with the *yin*. The *yin qiao* has the specific function of enabling the *yin* to ascend – especially the *yin* and essences from the kidneys. It takes the *yin* right up to the top of the body, to the eyes and the brain. It is responsible for irrigation and the irrigation is distributed by this springing up movement.

The *qiao* movement comes before the division into *yin* and *yang*, and the *qiao* quality has two aspects. In this presentation in the Nanjing, the *yang* is connected with the gallbladder and the wind. But the *yin* also has the ability to rise up; it ascends to the pharynx and connects with the *chong mai*. We have seen that the *yin qiao* can be coupled with the *ren mai*, but that is not mentioned here; it is a different kind of relationship. The *chong mai* is called the sea of blood and the sea of the *jing mai*, and there is a manifestation of both *ren mai* and *chong mai* at the pharynx. So this represents the reunion of the *yin qiao mai* with the *yin* power of the extraordinary meridians shown first in the *ren mai* and then through some of the *yin* functions of the *chong mai*, which we have seen to be the sea of blood, the sea of the *jing mai*, and to be responsible for the irrigation of the small and great valleys. This text connects the *yin qiao* with this same quality of vitality.

The extraordinary meridians are always concerned with the development of the unfolding of *yin* and *yang*, of water and fire, essences and *qi*. The *qiao mai* are not only concerned with this basic organization, but also with a movement, an impetus which creates the ability to rise up. And of course if they control and regulate the ascending movement, they must also control and regulate the descending movement.

Chong mai and *ren mai* also penetrate the face, the *chong mai* inside the nose, the *ren mai* the area just below the eyes, so they ensure the complete irrigation or moistening of the face and provide the basic pattern for the ascending movement of the *jin ye* (津 液), allowing the moistening and irrigation of the orifices of the face, the brain and so on. This moistening and irrigating quality maintains and nourishes the muscles, which is very important in the pathology of the *qiao mai*. The muscles must always have sufficient irrigation coupled with good strength and movement. If there is not a good balance between both, there may be contractions and many other possible pathologies.

It is obvious that because there are two malleoli on both legs, there are two *yin qiao* and two *yang qiao*, and therefore they provide the first differentiation between right and left within the extraordinary meridians. But what do we mean by the right and the left? It is not only the right part and the left part, but also all the movement and circulation made by the left and the right – the ascending and the descending movements.

Claude Larre: Right and left are locations, but the reason why the Chinese designate right and left with ascending and descending is because the left is the position of the rising sun, the right of the setting sun. Life rises with the rising sun, and sets with the setting sun. It is not necessary to elaborate more than that, but it is important to remember that when the Chinese are talking about left and right they always assume these connections with the movement of the sun which is the same within ourselves as in the universe.

Elisabeth Rochat: The malleolus is a very important area for the pathways of the meridians of the foot. At the internal malleolus, there are the three *yin* meridians of the foot, the three muscular meridians of the three *yin* of the foot, and also the *luo* of the kidneys and liver. At the external malleolus there are the bladder and gallbladder meridians, their muscular meridians and the three *luo* of the bladder, gallbladder and stomach. At the middle of the heel, there is a branch of the kidney meridian, but also the *luo* of the kidneys. At the external part of the heel there is the muscular meridian of the bladder. We can begin to see that there is a special relationship between the *qiao mai* and the bladder and kidney meridians.

According to Li Shizhen:

'The *yang qiao* (陽 蹻) detaches (*bie* 別) from the *tai yang* of the foot. This *mai* surges from the middle of the heel. It emerges under the external malleolus, at the point *shen mai* (申 脈 Bl 62) on the *tai yang* of the foot. At the level of the back of the malleolus, it turns around the heel to root itself (*ben* 本) at *pu can* (僕 參 Bl 61). It rises directly, running over the external face of the thigh, runs over the back of the ribs and rises to the top of the back. It meets the *tai yang* of the hand at *nao yu* (臑 俞 SI 10). It rises up on the external side of the shoulder and above the scapula and meets the *yang ming* of the hand at *jian yu* (LI 15). It rises to *ren ying* (人 迎 St 9), and surrounds the corners of the mouth. It meets with the *yang ming* of the hand and foot and *ren mai* at *di cang* (地 倉 St 4). Together with the *yang ming* of the foot it rises to *ju liao* (巨 髎 St 3). It meets once more with *ren mai* at *cheng qi* (承 泣 St 1). It reaches the internal corner of the eye where there is a meeting of the five *mai*: *tai yang* of the hand and foot, *yang ming* of the foot, *yin qiao* and *yang qiao*, at *jing ming* (睛 明 Bl 1). From *jing ming* it rises and penetrates the hairline, it descends behind the ear, penetrates *feng chi* (風 池 GB 20) where it ends. In all 22 points.'

'The *yin qiao* (陰 蹻) detaches (*bie* 別) from the *shao yin* of the foot. Together with the *shao yin*, it runs along the internal malleolus under the point *zhao hai* (照 海 Ki 6). It rises two *cun* above the internal malleolus to make *jiao jin* (交 信 Ki 8) its reserve, *xi* (郗 *xi* cleft point), then it rises directly, running over the anterior internal face of the thigh and penetrates the *yin* (sexual organ). It rises, running through the thorax and penetrates *que pen* (缺 盆 St 12), it rises, coming out in front of *ren ying* (人 迎 St 9). It reaches the larynx, with which it makes an exchange, *jiao* (交) and links with *chong mai*. It penetrates the internal side of the malar bone, it rises to take a dependent relation with the internal corner of the eye, where there is a meeting of the five *mai*: *tai yang* of the hand and foot, *yang ming* of the foot, *yang qiao* and *yin qiao* at *jing ming* (睛 明 Bl 1). In all eight points.'

The description of the pathways by Li Shizhen stresses the difference between the *yin* and the *yang qiao*. The *yin qiao* runs over the anterior internal side of the thigh and penetrates the *yin*, the genitals. The use of this particular term for the genitals (*yin* 陰) emphasizes the concentration of *yin* in the lower abdomen and the function of the kidneys on the *yin* of the body – essences, fluids etc. The *yin qiao mai* has a very important function in this area. It then runs through the thorax, making a connection between the *yin* of the lower heater and that of the upper heater, penetrating *que pen* (缺 盆 St 12), which is the meeting point of many pathways and currents of the vital circulation. It rises to *ren ying* (人 迎 St 9) making a strong connection with the stomach meridian. Li Shizhen repeats the exchange and connection with *chong mai* which is given in the Nanjing, stressing the internal aspect of the body. Then there is the junction with *jing ming* (睛 明 Bl 1) at the inner canthus of the eye. Li Shizhen describes a junction of the two *qiao mai* at *jing ming*, which is also seen in Lingshu chapter 17.

Jing ming (睛 明) suggests both light and the illumination that comes from a good irrigation by the essences. *Jing* is usually used for the pupil of the eye, but here it also refers to the gathering of the essences (*jing* 精) of the five *zang* and the six *fu*, as is often expressed in the texts, for example Lingshu 80 and Suwen 81. This is another way to show how the vitality is brought to the upper orifices and to the brain by the *qiao mai*.

In the Nanjing we saw their common origin in the middle of the heel. The *yin qiao* goes through the inner part of the trunk, the *yang qiao* more to the back and at the top of the back meeting with the *tai yang* of the hand (small intestine meridian) and the *shao yang* of the foot (gallbladder meridian). So there is a double trajectory of the *qiao*, one on the inner *yin* part of the body, which goes through the lower abdomen and the chest, making contact with *chong mai*, and another trajectory on the *yang* part, enveloping the back and the external part of the body. There is a conjunction of the effort of the *qiao mai* at the eyes, and we will see the effect of all these meetings with the eyes and the brain in their function and pathology.

The *yin* and *yang qiao* give the rhythm of *yin* and *yang* to each moment of life; the equilibrium between essences and *qi*, blood and *qi*, but also the good balance with *yin* and *yang* in our surroundings – night and day for example. That and other aspects of the function of the *qiao mai* are seen in the area of the eyes.

Commentaries on the Nanjing and other texts suggest that the *zang* and the innermost aspects of the body are irrigated by the *yin qiao mai*, and the *fu* are watered by the *yang qiao mai*. This is just another way to show the total impregnation in the rising up movement of the *yin* and *yang* of the body. This could be interpreted as the *zang* and the *fu*, or the inner and outer parts of the body, or the front and the back – all interpretations are possible, because the main function of the *qiao mai* is to rule the exchanges and to create equilibrium between the *yin* and the *yang* at every level.

Their conjunction at Bladder 1 completes the circle. The first model of circulation between *yin* and *yang* is made with *ren mai* and *du mai*, which envelope and encircle the primary structure of the body. Here with the *qiao mai*, which are of course linked with *ren mai* and *du mai*, we have a larger circle from the feet to the top of the head, and also a circle enveloping inner and outer at each level of the body. They unite at the eyes in order to begin the next cycle. The circulation of *wei qi* begins at the eyes, it envelopes all the external parts of the body during the day and regulates the innermost parts during the night. This is an example of the effect of the circulation of the *qiao mai*.

The anchoring of *yin* and *yang qiao mai* at the heel, and

at the malleolus with the kidney and bladder meridians, is usually made at Kidney 6 and Bladder 62. The study of the names of these points can give us an idea of the mutual exchange and penetration of the two *qiao mai.*

Bladder 62 *shen mai* 申脈

Shen (申) is the name of the ninth of the twelve earthly branches, and it corresponds to the time of the afternoon between three and five o'clock. That is quite interesting because it is the time of the day when *yin* begins to manifest. The character suggests the idea of starting again, doubling up in order to express something. It also has the meaning of to be at ease, a kind of stretching. If we add the radical for a human being (伸) it means to stretch, but also to straighten up, with a feeling of expansion and extension. If you add the character mouth (呻) it is a deep sigh: a deep long aspiration coming from the lower abdomen in the area of the kidneys and lower heater in order to restore expansion to a blockage in respiration – for example, if there is a blockage in the thorax hampering respiration.

Another name for this point is *yang qiao,* because it is the anchoring point of the *yang qiao.*

The name of this point is explained by its relationship to the *yang qiao mai,* which is able to rise, expand and extend its influence for the benefit for the whole body, especially the *yang,* because this character also has the meaning of 'to distribute benevolence'. This is seen particularly in the Book of Odes.

According to some interpretations the name also indicates pathology, for example with the ability to contract but not to stretch. This is a later interpretation made through the usual pathology of the *qiao mai*, but this character to extend, to propagate, to stretch, also has the technical meaning in medicine of extension as opposed to flexion. All the musculature is involved here.

Kidney 6 *zhao hai* 照 海

Hai (海) is the sea, and has the radical for water on the left. *Zhao* (照) is to light, to illuminate and to reflect something, as if in a mirror, and has the fire radical underneath. There is something in the name of this point that suggests both fire and water. Kidney 2 (*ran gu* 然 谷) is the fire element point, but at Kidney 6 there is a meeting of fire and water. This is the meaning of its name – the reflecting power of the light on a sea of water. The interpretation is that fire and water are reflecting one another to combine the *yin* and *yang* of the kidneys and to reflect the unity of the fire and water of *ming men*. It is very interesting that at this point where the *yin qiao* rises there is a communion between water and fire; the power of the fire being able to raise up the qualities of the water. This alliance creates a balance between the *yin* and the *yang* aspects of life. If we look at the movement of the kidney meridian at the malleolus there is a doubling back, but after this point the meridian is able to rise up.

So *zhao hai* expresses the unity of water and fire in the kidneys, but also the relationship with the origin, and the power of the origin. There are many commentaries on this point discussing the relationship with authentic *yang* which is able to illuminate authentic *yin* and so on. Another name for the point is *yin qiao*.

Shen mai is an expression of elevation and stretching, but it also referred to the time of day when the *yang* welcomes the *yin*. This specific time of the day when the *yin* appears (3 - 5 pm) is also the time of the most powerful activity of the bladder meridian, and of course the point *shen mai* is on the bladder meridian. These two names are very interesting in that each shows one side welcoming the other. With *shen mai* the *yang* is welcoming the *yin*, and here in *zhao hai*, the *yin* is accepting the *yang*, allowing the *yang* to illuminate and motivate while remaining within the quality of *yin* and water; like the clarity of a mirror reflecting through the water.

It is the ability of *yin qiao mai* to accept the *yang* and for *yang qiao mai* to accept the *yin*, which is expressed in these two points and the result is visible at eyes, where their conjunction is made and the work of the two meridians has its effective.

In other classical texts, other points are mentioned in relation to the *qiao mai*. Bladder 59 (*fu yang* 附 陽), Gallbladder 29 (*ju liao* 居 髎), Du 16 (*feng fu* 風 府) for the *yang qiao* and for the *yin qiao*, Kidney 2 (*ran gu* 然 谷). This does not necessarily mean that the *yin qiao* begins at *ran gu* but rather implies the power of the fire and the beginning of this ability to rise that is seen at Kidney 2.

Yin qiao has a very strong link with the kidney meridian, and the *yang qiao* links with all the *yang* meridians except the *shao yang* of the hand, the triple heater meridian. No points of the triple heater meridian are given in the trajectory of the *yang qiao mai*.

LINGSHU CHAPTER 17

Elisabeth Rochat: The first part of this chapter is a presentation of the complete length of the meridians in the human body. The calculation is made by adding the length of the twelve main meridians and the *du mai* and *ren mai*. In these calculations the *yin qiao mai* is added for women, the *yang qiao mai* for men. There is then an explanation of the relationship between the five *zang* and the upper orifices. Just after that the Emperor asks this question:

'Huangdi: From where does this *qiao mai* arise, and where does it stop? How is its *qi* concerned with nourishing and watering?

'Qi Bo: *Qiao* detaches from the *shao yin,* rising at the back of *ran gu* (Ki 2 然谷). It rises over the inner malleolus and ascends following the internal part of the thigh, penetrating the *yin* (sexual organs). It rises following the inner part of the chest and enters *que pen* (St 12 缺盆). It exits in front of *ren ying* (St 9 人迎). It enters below the eyes and has a *shu* (屬 dependent, belonging) relationship with the inner corner of the eyes, where it makes a junction with *tai yang* and *yang qiao* and continues to rise. There is an association of *qi* for mutual exchange and the eyes are moistened. If the *qi* is unable to provide nutrition, the eyes cannot close.

'Huangdi asks: If *qi* is circulating only in the five *zang* and is not nourishing the six *fu*, why is that?

'Qi Bo replies: As for the *qi*, it is impossible for it not to circulate. It is like water flowing; like the sun and the moon circulating unceasingly. The *yin mai* nourishes the *yin*, the *yang mai* gives splendour to the *yang*. It is like a circle without end, perpetually unrolling; when it is finished it begins again. This *qi* flowing with a great abundance irrigates and waters the five *zang* in the interior, and in the exterior humidifies and moistens the pores and skin.'

The *yin qiao* is presented as a detachment (*bie* 別) from the kidney meridian. One important point is that emphasis is given to the nutritive or *yin* aspect of the circulation. At the same time there is the idea of a kind of splendour. This splendour is to act in such a way that the magnificent effects of the vitality can be seen in each of the *zangfu*, each orifice and part of the body; they are all well irrigated, nourished and maintained by the essences. The character *rong* (榮 splendour) is used several times in this text.

This is particularly relevant to the conjunction of the *qiao mai* at the eyes, at *jing ming* (晴 明 Bl 1). This is the commanding area for the defensive *qi*, and here, through the *qiao mai*, we can also see the rising movement of the other aspect of the *qi*, the nutritive *qi*, the fluids and essences, in a dual relationship with the defensive *qi*. This is another way to present what was certainly considered the main function of the *qiao* in ancient times, this perpetual conjunction of *yin* and *yang*, and a conjunction of the nutritive and the defensive *qi*. The relationship of the *qiao mai* with the defensive *qi* is seen in other chapters, here there is an obvious relationship with the nutritive *qi*.

The beginning the text just says *qiao mai*. But it says that at the eyes it has a conjunction with *tai yang* and *yang qiao*, so here it is especially the *yin qiao mai*, but more particularly the importance of the *qiao* function for the *yin*. The point *ran gu* (然 谷 Ki 2) is mentioned perhaps to emphasize the power of the fire and the *yang* in giving the *yin* the possibility to rise. The pathway after that is nearly the same as in the Li Shizhen text.

At the end of the first section we see that if this all works well the eyes can open and close; we are able to follow the natural rhythm of *yin* and *yang* in the universe through day and night. This is the first mention of the relationship with *wei qi* (衛 氣), the defensive *qi*, which is in charge of the manifestation of the rhythms of day and night within human life, for example the opening and closing of the eyes. But this text explains that this is only possible if the muscles are well moistened. If the muscles are contracted, you physically cannot close your eyes. And if there is not a good balance between *yin* and *yang*, water and fire, in the body, there may be insomnia or somnolence due to a disturbance of the eyes.

Another commentator, Zhang Zicong, has a very good explanation of this. He says that the Emperor's question is relating to *qi* and to nutrition and fluids. This is the reason why Qi Bo answers with *yin qiao*. It is through the *yin qiao* and the close relationship between *yin qiao* and the kidneys and the kidney meridian that there is sufficient nutritive power for the irrigation of the five *zang*. And there is also a relationship between the irrigation of the five *zang* with the spirit of the heart and the formation of the blood.

This commentator also said that as the *qi* of *yin* and *yang qiao* are joined together, the exterior and interior are in an exchange and relationship and inter-penetrate one another. This is the idea of a *luo* relationship, and the *qiao mai* are a prototype of the *luo* function. Behind the interior and exterior relationship are the *ying* (營) and the *wei* (衛), nutrition and defence. Nutrition is effective in the interior and the defence more on the exterior.

The second part of Qi Bo's answer, with reference to the sun and the moon and the cycles of the body, explains the continuity of the circulation as a circle without end. The revolving movement is in all directions, ascending and descending; here there is a rising movement of the *yin*, of essences and nutrition, and perhaps this is in contrast with the presentation of the trajectory of the defensive *qi* given in Lingshu 76, which descends from the eyes.

All parts of the body are irrigated by the *qiao mai*; the *zang* and *fu* and all the internal viscera, and all the parts of the body right up to the *cou li* (腠 理), the most external structures of the body. All this is well nourished and maintained. The images of the sun and the moon are very rich and suggest all the various rhythms of life, the regular course of the sun as well as the transformation of the moon and all possible effects and correspondences in the body, including the ability to adapt the equilibrium of blood and *qi*, *yin* and *yang*.

The Emperor continues and says:

> '*Qiao mai*, they are *yin* and *yang*. But which *mai* is included in the calculation (*shu* 數)?'

Shu (數) is to count, it is a number or a calculation. But also it is to arrive through calculation at a good and effective arrangement of numbers, for example to arrive at a good method of treatment. All these meanings are included here. Qi Bo replies:

> 'For men the *shu* is *yang*, for women the *shu* is *yin*.'

The *shu* becomes part of the calculation of the length of the meridian system and what is not the *shu* is the *luo*. This suggests that if the *qiao mai* are the first separation within the organism, they also represent the first separation of *yin* and *yang* within the male and female species, and they provide one way to understand the difference in the manifestation of the equilibrium between blood and *qi* in men and women. That is why for men, when calculating the total length of the *mai* we count the *yang qiao mai*, which is called the meridian, because the *yang* is the norm for men. It is the opposite for women. As a result of this, when you treat through the *qiao mai* it is different for men and women.

In treating the *qiao* through the two points Kidney 6 and Bladder 62, we have to be aware of the sex of the patient. This is part of a method of treatment according to the Neijing. The man is ruled more by the *yang* and the *qi*, the woman by the *yin* and the blood. So here again this *luo* relationship is linked with the *qiao mai*. It is rather complicated and I am not sure whether it is practically useful. It is possibly something that belonged to a particular school in ancient times.

Commenting on this Zhong Zicong says:

'The *yin qiao mai* rise from the foot corresponding to the rising of the *qi* of the earth. This is the reason why women have the addition (*shu* 數) of the *yin qiao*. The *yin qiao* belongs to the inner corner of the eye, where it makes a junction with the *yang qiao* and rises up. The *yang qiao* receives the *qi* of the *yin qiao* and from the border of the hair continues and descends down to the foot corresponding to the descending movement of the *qi* of heaven. That is the reason why the number (*shu* 數) of men is given by the *yang qiao*.'

This is a specific way to explain the perpetual movement of ascending and descending – the ascending movement of the *yin* and the descending movement of the *yang* – which is similar to certain presentations of the *du mai* and *ren mai*. The rising up of the *qi* coming from the earth and the descending movement of the *qi* coming from heaven; *yin* and *yang*. There is always this kind of exchange and continual reversal. The *yang* continually expands and rises up but at the same time it is like the lungs which have descending movement in order to irrigate and impregnate the whole body. And it is the reverse for the *yin*.

That is an important aspect of the *qiao mai*. The *yin qiao mai* allows the essences of the water of the *shao yin*, kidney meridian, to be in free communication with the *yang qiao*. The *yang qiao mai* allows the *qi* of *tai yang*, bladder meridian, to be in free communication with the *yin qiao*. This is the same for male and female.

THE QIAO MAI IN OTHER TEXTS

Quoting an ancient text Zhang Zicong says:

> '*Tai yang* and *shao yin* of the foot are the source from which blood and *qi*, *yin* and *yang* are originally produced. *Yin qiao mai* and *yang qiao mai* master the free communication of *yin* and *yang*. Blood and *qi* from below rise and have an exchange and mutual connection at the eyes.'

Lingshu chapter 21 gives a description of *tai yang* of the foot, which takes a *shu* (belonging) relationship with the root of the eye. It continues:

> '...This pathway enters the brain and there is a separation between *yin qiao* and *yang qiao*. *Yin* and *yang* meet together (*jiao* 交).'

Jiao is an exchange where the *yang* penetrates the *yin* and the *yin* exits to the *yang*. This meeting and exchange takes place at the inner corner of the eyes. When the *yang qi* increase in power, the eyes open, when the *yin qi* increase in power the eyes close.

At the inner corner of the eyes we see the external effect of a mechanism that takes place within the depths of the brain. The brain is also linked with the kidneys and is the meeting place of the essences and marrow, but it is entirely impregnated and illuminated by the *qi* coming through all the *yang* meridians, and also by the presence of the spirits. This is how the brain is able to work well and enable the upper orifices, particularly the eyes, to function well.

The eyes are sometimes called the gates of destiny (*ming men* 命 門, because at the eyes there is a meeting of essences coming from the five *zang* and the six *fu*. This text fits very well with Lingshu chapter 17 on the rising up of essences and fluids. The eyes are the meeting place of the essences, but they are also the meeting place of all the *yang* meridians and the dwelling place and reception for the expression of the spirits – the eyes being the messenger and expression of the depths of the heart. The relationship between spirit and the eyes is not merely symbolic – the eyes are the actual location of this function. All the rhythms of nutritive and defensive *qi* are linked to this area and to the brain, the function of *du mai* and the bladder meridian and so on. That is why the eyes are also called the gate of life or life destiny, (*ming men* 命 門); they are the visible manifestation of the ability to manage vitality, the conjunction of *yin* and *yang* and the expression of the spirits.

Another interesting thing in this text is that it does not describe quite the same movement. *Yin* and *yang* complete their own movement and turn to one another, the *yang* penetrating the *yin*. This is a way to describe the defensive *qi* entering into the depths of the body at night, and penetrating into the *yin*. The other movement is the development within the *yin* which goes out to the *yang* and gives the nourishment necessary for everyday life to the external parts of the body, for example, the limbs and the orifices. If this relationship is good, one enriches the other. When the *yin* becomes weak, for example at dawn, there is a movement of the *qi* and blood towards the exterior, the eyes open and the limbs move. This is the normal movement. When the *yang qi* is powerful, the *yin* goes out to the *yang*. This enables the opening of the eyes. When the *yin qi* increases in power the *yang* is able to enter the *yin*, and the eyes close.

Later chapters of the Lingshu describe the relationship of the *qiao mai* with the rhythms of sleeping and waking and to the circulation of the *wei qi*, the defensive *qi*. Chapter 76 describes the circulation of the *wei qi*. By diffusion through the *yang* meridians, the *wei qi* is directed towards the exterior for movement and communication with the exterior.

The last trajectory is through the *yang ming* of foot and hand (stomach and large intestine meridians) to the teeth. The text then says that the *wei qi* goes to the 'heart of the foot' and exits under the inner malleolus, at the area of the *shao yin* of the foot (kidney meridian). This is of course the place of the *yin qiao mai*. There is then a meeting at the eyes which makes one circuit. There are 25 circuits during the day.

It is important to pay attention to the reality of this circulation and to understand the rhythms underlying it. If we think of the defensive *qi* as something substantial flowing inside one meridian, then another and then through the *yin qiao mai* going up to the eyes and so on, this does not give a true representation of this mechanism. This is one circulation among several others. There may be all kinds of variations due to age, to the phases of the moon, to external influences of cold and heat and so on. This description is rather to indicate one of the great rhythms of life, and the way in which to treat a deficiency of this rhythm – through the *qiao mai*, through the *yang* meridians or through the *zang*, depending where the deficiency in the rhythm occurs.

In this chapter, the *yin qiao*, which was also mentioned in Lingshu chapter 17 as the vector for the rising up of essences and fluids and nutritive power, is also linked with the trajectory of the defensive *qi*. It is also through the *yin qiao* that there is a passage to the kidneys at night to keep the defensive *qi* inside the body. If this is not working well, there may be all kinds of symptoms linked to an imbalance between the *yin* and the *yang*, such as night sweating.

In Lingshu chapter 71 there is a triple presentation of the ancestral *qi* (*zong qi* 宗 氣) accumulated in the middle of the chest, the nutritive *qi* (*ying qi* 營 氣) and finally of the defensive *qi* (*wei qi* 衛 氣). It says that the defensive *qi* 'exits with the rapidity and agility of a very brave and fierce chief'. The defensive *qi* is always described in this way as very brave, fierce and full of courage. And the character *qiao* has a similar meaning of this kind of rapidity and proud courage. The *wei qi* circulates first to the four extremities, to the mass of flesh and all the cracks and crevices in the layers of the skin. During the day it circulates in the *yang* and at night it circulates in the *yin*. It is always from the area of the *shao yin* of the foot (kidney meridian) that it is able to circulate through the five *zang* and the six *fu*.

The text then mentions a situation of *jue qi* (厥 氣), which is a situation where the *qi* are unable to reach their area of responsibility, creating an empty space and a counter-current of perverse energy which flows in to fill the empty space. If this situation occurs in the five *zang* and six *fu*, the defensive *qi* is only able to defend the exterior and circulate in the *yang*, but is unable to enter the *yin*. Circulating only in the *yang*, there is an increase of the power of the *yang qi*. If the *yang qi* increases in power, which here is a pathological overflowing, the *yang qiao* is congested (*man* 滿). If all the *yang* meridians and the superficial pathways of the body, for instance the *luo*, are congested with a pathological fullness, the *yang qiao* will be congested. This is because not only one pathway is involved, but it is a general condition of the *yang*.

If the *jue* generates a counter-current, the *yang* is unable to enter the *yin* and that is the particular pathology of the *qiao*: there is no communication or exchange between *yin* and *yang*. If the *yang qiao* is congested, there is no possibility for the *yang qiao* or the defensive *qi* to enter the *yin*. And by the same mechanism, if the *yin* is empty, the inward movement is too weak, and *wei qi* cannot enrich the power of the *yin* part of the body. This is the reason why the eyes cannot close. The eyes manifest the weakness of the mutual exchange of *yin* and *yang*, essences and *qi* and so on. It is also because of the imbalance in sleeping and waking that there is weakness of the balance of the *zang* themselves.

Later in the text Huangdi asks what the treatment should be. Qi Bo replies:

> 'Tonify where there is deficiency and disperse where there is excess, to harmonize emptiness and fullness in order to restore free communication of all the pathways and to expel the perverse. When the *yin* and the *yang* are again in free communication there is sleep.'

Lingshu chapter 80 presents the same idea. At the beginning of the chapter there is this sentence:

> 'The essences and *qi* from the five *zang* and the six *fu* rise to pool in the eyes and make essence (*jing* 精).'

This is also the ability to see. The eyes cannot express the light of life without this conjunction of pure essences and *qi* from the five *zang* and the six *fu*. Later in the same chapter:

'The eyes are the essences of the five *zang* and the six *fu*, the permanent place for nutrition and defence; for the *hun* as well as the *po*. It is the place where *shen* and *qi* are produced. ...When *yin* and *yang* are well connected and in an harmonious relationship there is the phenomenon called *jing ming* (精 明).'

This is the *jing* (精) of essences and the *ming* (明) of illumination. Illumination is the radiance of life coming from the spirits and from the root of life. It is not only a play of words, it is a play with the reality of communication at this area. If the eyes are capable of all these phenomena it is because they are a very special place where all the aspects of life come together and manifest themselves. *Jing ming* is a way to express the mechanisms necessary for the subtle workings of the upper orifices. There must be essences, which are brought through the strength of the *qi*, and illumination coming from the spirits – not only to have good sight but to have sight with discernment. The spirits must be present and the heart must be present in all the orifices – especially the very subtle orifices of the eyes and the ears. This conjunction is all part of the function of the *qiao mai*.

The text continues saying that the eyes are the messenger of the heart and that the heart is the dwelling place of the spirits. Then there is a presentation of the great pattern for insomnia and sleepiness, which is the same as in chapter 71. This is a very important part of the pathology of the *qiao mai*.

When the defensive *qi* is unable to enter the *yin* but stays continuously in the *yang*, the *yang qi* is congested. If the *yang qi* is congested, the *yang qiao* increases its power and is unable to enter the *yin*. Consequently the *yin qi* are empty and the eyes are unable to close. Conversely, when the defensive *qi* stays in the *yin* and is unable to circulate in the *yang* the *yin qi* increases its power. When the *yin qi* increases its power, the *yin qiao* is congested and is unable to penetrate into the *yang*. The *yang qi* is empty and the eyes remain closed.

PATHOLOGY OF THE QIAO MAI

Nanjing difficulty 29:

> 'When *yin qiao* gives rise to illnesses, the *yang* is relaxed or loosened (*huan* 緩) and the *yin* is tense (*ji* 急). When *yang qiao* gives rise to illness, the *yin* is relaxed or loosened (*huan* 緩) and the *yang* is tense (*ji* 急).'

There is an obvious parallel here between the symptoms of the *yin* and *yang qiao mai*. We see this in other texts – the same symptoms reversed for the *yin* and *yang qiao mai*. The *wei mai* do not have the same pattern, it is quite different, but this kind of parallel is very common for the *qiao mai*. There are two characters here, one is *huan* (緩) which means loose, and the other is *ji* (急). *Huan* can have positive meanings in other contexts but generally *ji* has the negative meaning of cramped, and it can be used for muscular contractions. *Huan* means to be loose or without enough tension to ensure circulation and communication. The text can be interpreted in two ways depending on whether you choose the normal or the pathological meaning of this character *huan*.

The symptoms are presented as a couple; when the *yang* is in this situation of cramps, the *yin* is relaxed and loose, without strength and movement, because here there is not enough *yin* and irrigation. There is separation of *yin* and *yang* and blood and *qi* instead of cooperation. As it is the pathology of the *qiao mai* it is not related to a particular area of the body.

There may be congestion in the *yang*, and as a consequence an emptiness in the *yin* through the mechanism of the *yin qiao*. Or there may be congestion of the *yin qiao* causing congestion in all the *yin* circulation with contractions in the *yin qiao*, and a lack of strength in all the *yang* circulation.

Some commentators say that if the *yin qiao* is affected first, if it is congested or in pathological fullness, the symptom of cold will be predominant, and if the *yang qiao* is in this state of fullness, tension and congestion, the symptoms of heat and agitation will be predominant.

That brings us to another kind of pathology linked with the *qiao mai*, the two sides of fury and madness, agitation and inertia, which are also effects of this lack of communication between *yin* and *yang*; the bolting of the *yang* or the overflowing of the *yin*. Classically, fury is a doubling of the *yang*, and dementia with prostration is a doubling of the *yin*. Another symptom often linked with dementia or fury is convulsions. With these convulsions there are symptoms of contraction or alternating contraction and cramps which are part of the pathology of the *qiao mai*.

Suwen chapter 62:

'When there is pain but one is unable to locate it, the best thing is (to treat) the two *qiao*.'

The character used for two is *liang* (兩) which means a couple or a pair. The character shows two together under the same yoke, which is a good representation of the *qiao mai*. Some commentators see a reference here to all kinds of blockage due to damp, because in this case it is very difficult to localize the pain.

The commentator Wu Kun says if the two *qiao mai* are related to the kidney and bladder meridians, they are also related to cold and to water. And the best way to treat is by tonification or moxibustion in case of dampness due to cold and excess water in the body. But this is a particular interpretation.

The general interpretation is that if the two *qiao mai* control the general relationship of the equilibrium of each muscle inside the body and each mass of flesh, they are always acting to restore good communication. The obvious points are *shen mai* (Bl 62) and *shao hai* (Ki 6) and, according to many commentators, both together. This kind of pain may be very acute, or there may be a kind of numbness and paralysis depending on the case.

The same idea is found in Lingshu chapter 73, with nearly the same words:

'If one is unable to localize the pain one needles the two qiao, (*liang qiao* 兩 蹻) below. If one needles the *yin* for a man and the *yang* for a woman, one does something forbidden to a practitioner of a high level.'

This is an application of the theory that the *yang qiao* is strong within men and able to regulate both the *qiao mai,* while the *yin qiao* is strong within women and able to regulate both the *qiao mai.* It is more effective to treat where there is strength, where there is the best response and the best reception. Some commentators suggest applying moxa to these two points of *yin* and *yang qiao mai.* This kind of pain is often linked to cold and damp which is the reason why moxibustion is the best treatment.

The problem with this text is that some commentators interpret it in the opposite way, saying that you must treat the *yin* in men and the *yang* in women. I don't think that it is very important. It is probably safer to treat both, as it says in the commentary on chapter 62 of the Suwen! Of course we may use Kidney 6 and Bladder 62 together. It is also possible to tonify Kidney 6 and disperse Bladder 62, or the opposite, which is a common way to use these points. It depends on the diagnosis and also on the time of day. You can use moxa on the *yang qiao mai* treating a patient in the morning for instance. This is a good example of the time of the treatment being of great importance, especially in the treatment of insomnia. You can change the treatment according to the time of day.

This non-communication between *yin* and *yang* is the first aspect of the pathology of the *qiao mai*. Another aspect of the pathology is related to the eyes, and particularly pain and redness in the eyes. Here the treatment is on the *qiao mai*, as we can see in Lingshu chapter 23:

'When there is redness and pain at the middle of the eyes, beginning from the inner corner of the eyes, one needles the *yin qiao*.'

The commentators indicate that treatment is to tonify the point *zhao hai* (Ki 6). This is a situation of non-communication between the *yin* and the *yang*, between the lower and upper part of the organism. Because there is redness, there is too much *yang* at the eyes, and you must tonify the rising power of the *yin* to balance that. There is a similar description in Suwen chapter 63:

'When perverse *qi* are lodged in the *yang qiao mai*, that causes pain in the eye which begins from the internal corner of the eye. One needles half a *cun* under the external malleolus. Each time one makes two insertions. For the left, one takes the right, for the right one takes the left. In the time it takes to walk ten *li*, it is over.'

This is another interesting example. This chapter is about *miu* (繆) puncture. *Miu* puncture is a special kind of treatment on the *luo* used when the disease is located in the *luo* and has not yet reached the main meridians. You needle the points at the extremities, the *jing* well points, to evacuate the perverse *qi*. In the needling technique there is usually a crossing between left and right. If the symptoms are on the right, treatment is often on the left side, in order to make use of the rapidity and facility of circulation proper to the *luo*. This is another example of the role of the *qiao mai* as a kind of rapidity of communication and the ability to move from the right to the left and from the left to the right. This relationship of left and right is also one of the qualities of the *qiao mai*, which is another similarity with the *luo* function.

What in the Chinese is called *luo* refers not only to the twelve or fifteen great *luo*, they are just one particular network of relationships. In the area crossed by each meridian there is a provision, made by the meridian, of a complete network of circulation which is also called the *luo*. The *luo* spread throughout the territory of the main meridian with branches covering all the space. The *luo* are everywhere. If there are symptoms in the area under the authority of a particular meridian, but the perverse *qi* is not in the meridian itself but in the *luo*, you must treat with this quality which provides rapidity of movement. Because it is in this area that the *yang* quality of the defensive *qi* is found at the exterior of the meridian, and the ability to move and penetrate is the main quality of this *qi*.

This chapter of the Suwen describes many of these symptoms in its definition of *miu* puncture. A complete healing with one treatment can be assured within this short time because the perverse *qi* are superficial and in the *yang*, and especially at the upper part of the body where the *yang* expresses itself.

If there is pain in the eyes caused by tension within the connections of the eyes, and possibly dryness, disperse the excess of *yang*. Because it is not specifically in one meridian, and because it is at the level of the eyes, you can treat this superficial perversion by dispersion of this point of the *yang qiao* (Bl 62) – giving the instruction through the *yang qiao*, to the *yang* circulation in the *luo*. This is another way to see the relationship between the *qiao mai* and the *luo*.

Elisabeth Rochat: In Suwen 63 there are two examples of pain at the eyes related to the *yin* and *yang qiao*. Here we have to disperse, but when the symptoms are at a deeper level you must tonify the *yin*. This is a question which arises with the *qiao mai*. The pulses are probably the best way to decide which is the best treatment.

Li Shizhen sums up all the symptoms linked with the *qiao mai*. Particularly quoting from the Mai Jing, the Classic of the Pulse, he says that with the *yang qiao* there are pains in the back and in the lumbar area. There may also be convulsions with madness, in which the patient falls down, stiff, with a fear of wind and a possibility of hemiplegia, and also a kind of *bi* (痹) syndrome which has been going on for a very long time; paralysis, stiffness and inability to move.

For the *yin qiao* he also mentions convulsions with madness, and we have seen the distinction between the two, and also *bi* (痹) syndrome with pain in the *yin*, the sexual organs. It is also said that in the case of *yin* disease, fullness of the *yin* and congestion of the *yin qiao*, the best treatment is to warm by using moxa on *zhao hai* (照 海 Ki 6) and *yang jiao* (陽 交

Gb 35). In the case of *yang* disease the treatment is to cool, and to needle *feng chi* (風 池 Gb 20) and *feng fu* (風 府 Du 16).

There is also some differentiation made according to the time of day when the symptoms occur. For instance for convulsions due to madness, if the convulsions occur during the day, the treatment is on the *yang qiao*, and if they occur during the night it is on the *yin qiao*.

If the *yang* is in excess at the eyes there may be insomnia, and if the *yin* is in excess at the eyes there may be sleepiness, but this is not exactly the case with cold and heat. For example there can be a fullness of heat causing loosening of the muscles and particularly of the muscles in the area of the eyes, when the muscles are unable to keep the eyes open. Conversely, cold in this area can cause a kind of contraction where it is painful and difficult to close the eyes. It is not exactly the same mechanism here.

The symptom of having the eyes open or closed is not as simple as it looks, it could be something other than insomnia or sleepiness. It can also be due to an attack on the muscles in this area. But there will always be other symptoms which make the diagnosis clearer. For example, the *yin qiao mai* may have a blockage of the *qi* at the pharynx, or there may be difficulty in urination, with pain in the bladder. For the *yang qiao mai* there may be stiffness, especially in the lumbar area and the back, swelling in the legs, fear of wind, spontaneous sweats, headache, or sweating on the head, with red painful eyes, or pain at the occiput, numbness and paralysis with cramps of the muscles and so on.

SUMMARY OF THE QIAO MAI

Elisabeth Rochat: The *qiao mai* represent the first division and repartition of *yin* and *yang*, with a common origin they affect the inner and the outer parts of the body, and meet not only at the inner corner of the eyes but also in the depths of the brain. Beginning in the middle of the heel they touch the power of the earth. They provide a kind of rooting in the earth, and take from the earth the strength to make all the earthly *qi*, the *yin*, essences, water and nutritive power rise up inside the body. Through their pathways, on the external and the internal parts of the body, on the left and on the right, they express the interpenetration and intercommunication of *yin* and *yang* at each level; with a particular relationship with defensive *qi* but also with nutritive *qi*.

All their connections are intra-systemic, within the same system, there is not yet a separation into two systems of *yin* and *yang*, but a double sense of *yin* and *yang* in the reality of the movement of *qiao* with all the up-surging spring of life. They are the first bilateral meridians, and they also resume the cyclic circulation through the whole movement of ascending and descending, the right and the left also representing this movement of going down and rising up.

Claude Larre: This seems very important to me from a logical point of view, because it shows that the *qiao mai* follow the same pattern as the *du mai* and *ren mai* which are circling in a closed cycle. They are just a development of the *du mai* and *ren mai*.

Elisabeth Rochat: This is the reason why they concern the *zang* and the *fu*, the *jing* (經) and the *luo*, the blood and the *qi*, and the relationship of interpenetration and good balance between one and the other. The relationship is not only in space, but also in time; not only the correct balance within any area of the body, but also the correct rhythm of time, for example day and night, and the way that one welcomes the other; the way that the *yin* is able to welcome the *yang*, and the *yang* welcomes the *yin* in both space and time.

Question: But the relationship with *ren mai* and *du mai* came at a later stage?

Elisabeth Rochat: I think that it is easy to understand why they made this kind of couple, though it is never actually referred to in the Neijing and the Nanjing.

Question: Is there a relationship made between the *yang qiao mai* and the liver? A lot of symptoms seem to be related.

Elisabeth Rochat: Any relationship that is made is because there is an analogy between the movement of the liver and the movement of *qiao*, this kind of uprising, which is also part of the nature of the gallbladder and liver. It is not by chance that the *yang qiao mai* finishes its trajectory at Gallbladder 20, and it is this point which is mentioned in the very short description in Nanjing difficulty 28. This is the point *feng chi*, which has a relationship to the wind, and to the gallbladder. The other point which is often mentioned is Gallbladder 29.

Some secondary texts give other points on the gallbladder meridian on the pathway of *yang qiao mai*, and in the treatment of *yang qiao mai*, for example Gallbladder 38 (*fu yang*). There are also relationships with the muscles, the muscular forces, and the pathology of the muscles, because the same movement is expressed by the *qiao mai* and by liver and gallbladder so we would expect to find similar symptoms.

Claude Larre: With reference to walking ten *li*, walking oils the muscles and bones and also warms the whole body. It may be that walking is a way to rebalance the *yang qiao mai*, because while walking the pain is diminishing and the whole body becomes balanced.

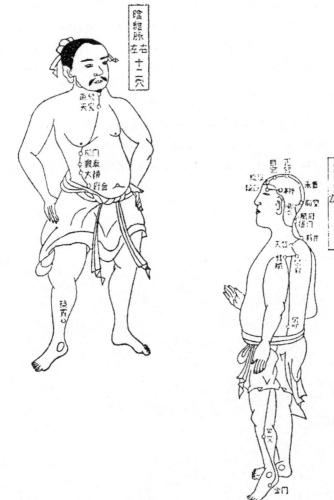

Yin and yang wei mai from the Neiwaigong tushuo

WEI MAI 維 脈

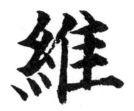

Claude Larre: This character *wei* (維) is not specific to Chinese medicine as such, it is a kind of rope, or the way that things are attached. The ten thousand beings are said to be attached (*wei* 維) between heaven and earth. It is not enough to say that they are simply placed between heaven and earth; it is through the essential influx and the receptive attitude of earth that things surge and have their place. It is through this attachment that they have a position and they have to be maintained in that position by some device. Things are maintained on earth at the four corners, that is where they are fixed. Stability on earth is expressed by four, and the link between things and beings and the earth is at the core of the concept of the *si wei* (四 維), the four attachments. How is something which is invisible able to be fixed and maintained in a particular place? We know that the ten thousand beings are alive, and so if there is something that can guarantee their stability, that something also has to be alive. So the *wei* is a device by which living beings are attached to earth.

Mythologically, the stability of earth is usually represented by the four feet of the tortoise – the tortoise being the sacred animal which gives fixity to everything everywhere between heaven and earth. And there must be a balance of *yin* and *yang*; if it were fixed by *yang* it would not be totally fixed, and if it were fixed by *yin* it would not be totally fixed. A living being has to be fixed through some *yin yang* device.

Dr Tim Gordon: The concept of the receptors for specific attachments is one of the most fundamental breakthroughs in modern biology and a great body of contemporary science was dependent on that discovery.

Claude Larre: The Chinese have made a progressively well-organized representation of the way things are made, produced, maintained and changed, and in general life it is the same, because the last change is death. When they are fixed, that fixity is made because of the necessity in life to have a place, and to have the means to make things fixed and stable. So the Western mind through chemistry, physics or biology would have the same preoccupation – it is the same world and the same mind when we come down to fundamentals. If two civilisations are able to give a good representation of the life of the universe, I think that the closer they come to the area where there is nothing to see, the more they will have the same ways of thinking. There may be more use of numbers in the Chinese thinking, because they have a very clear and very systematic presentation of numerology. The Western mind makes mathematical formula, which could never have happened with the Chinese because they give numbers a particular form of symbolism.

Elisabeth Rochat: The character for *wei* (維) is made with two parts, the left part is radical number 120, a thread of silk. This gives the image of a net, a network, and the ability to link or bind something. The character on the right is also part of the character for the triple heater, *san jiao* (三 焦) which has the fire radical in the lower part.

According to Wieger lesson 168 A, this represents a bird with a short tail, and suggests the linking and overlapping of the feathers on the body of a bird. This idea appears in many characters with this image, a bunch of bananas for example. Bananas are bunched together in the same way that the feathers of a bird fold over each other. It suggests a special kind of linking or attachment.

With the phonetic *zhui* (隹) and the thread of silk radical (糸) this character *wei* (維) means to tie, to hold fast; to attach with a rope, or to hold in a great net. The great net has a very firm and solid main string, which attaches all the smaller parts of the net. There are several other meanings which are more figurative.

The general meaning is to preserve something, because when something is maintained and held it is also preserved. You protect your boat by mooring it very firmly. And you preserve the kingdom by ruling with great laws and principles to ensure stability and to impress something on the mind and the behaviour of the people. This expression *si wei* (四 維), the four attachments, has a universal meaning as Father Larre said, but when speaking of the kingdom, it is a very common expression for the four fundamental virtues; it is to preserve the balance of the kingdom by being at the same time and in equal proportion benevolent, just and fair, to have balance between punishment and retribution and so on. The principle here is to have something very firm and secure as a reference point, and all kinds of people and things and behaviours can rely on these fixed things.

Claude Larre: The four cardinal virtues necessary for the stability of the state, are civility, justice, integrity and truth. Those four must make a totality. For every action there is not only a model but a way to carry it out. In the same way the four directions imply the regulation of everything and the expression *dong xi* (東 西) east and west, means everything under the sun, which rises in the east and sets in the west.

All this must be attached in the net. Laozi would say that the net of heaven is so large and so perfect that it covers and takes in everything without losing a single drop. In the particular case of the *wei mai*, we know that they are *yin* and *yang* and that they are four. But they are not concerned with the limbs as such, because this primary organization of the extraordinary meridians has more to do with the beginning of life where the limbs are not yet formed, and it takes time for a baby to be able to be physically active through the movement of the four limbs. So instead of the limbs, which are more characteristic of the ordinary meridians, the ancient Chinese would speak of the same principle of activity but at the level of the attachment of the *yin* and the *yang* in this particular life.

There is a kind of projection of life starting from the

fundamental organization of four by two, which is the eight
meridians, and when the organization is more complete
and the constitution of the individual has reached a certain
level, then all the activity is expressed by four multiplied by
three which gives us the twelve meridians. But since these
meridians are for normal practical life they are called the
ordinary meridians. The others are still there, and may be
used for specific reasons. We have the first four, which give a
kind of complete whole, then there are the two *qiao mai* with
this kind of upsurge of the vitality of life, and the two *wei*,
with a kind of firmness of attachment, linking for the same
stabilisation as the four directions which are the quality of *qi*
in the north, the west, the east and the south. Similarly the
four virtues are not for the individual, they are for the state.
They cover all the population.

Elisabeth Rochat: The term *si wei* may be used to describe
the four limbs, and it is by the four limbs that we come
into relationship with the exterior. The four limbs are for
movement and motion and the extremities of the four
limbs, with the *jing* well (井) points, communicate with the
qi coming from the exterior. We will find that again in the
pathology of the *wei mai*, especially the *yang wei mai*. The
four attachments provide a good balance on the left and the
right, above and below. If one of these four attachments and
moorings is not strong enough, the body will be in a state
of imbalance. It is the same thing in the country, if one of
the great principles ensuring the continuity of the kingdom
is too weak or too strong, there will be trouble. And it is
the same at the level of the cosmos; the four directions are
the reference points – attaching the world and allowing all

kinds of diverse and different *qi* and influences to have a good succession and an harmonious composition.

This character *wei* (維) for the *wei mai* contains all these ideas, and we can now begin to see the difference between the *qiao* and the *wei*. With the *qiao* the main idea was to put into motion, and rise up from the earth, with a community of *qi* within the *yin* and *yang qiao mai*, a perpetual interpenetration. With the *wei mai* it is more the way to maintain order because the *yin* and *yang*, and all kinds of *yin* and all kinds of *yang* in the body are maintained in a good proportion in order to compose an harmonious unity.

The usual interpretation of this character *wei* (維) by the commentators of the classics is to be able to hold firmly in the hands, to maintain and to support something. According to the commentators on the Nanjing, the *yang wei mai* is said to attach, to link, to tie and to support all the *yang*, and the same thing with the *yin* for the *yin wei mai*. They use this character *wei* like a verb, often adding another character which gives the idea that the *wei mai* are able to be present everywhere, like a net or like a great principle. The *yang wei* has this *wei* activity on all the *yang*. And the meaning here is like the virtue or the great rule, the ruling principle for the *yang* within the body. This is not the same as the *du mai*. The *du mai* is the first organization and appearance of the *yang* function in the body, in the lower abdomen, the heart, the spinal cord, the brain and the eyes. But now that the body is nearly complete and there are many more complex *yang* functions – all the meridians and *luo*, the exterior and interior with all the exchanges between the two. All this detailed *yang* function needs a unique rule. They need the main rope of the net to be held together and maintained. And the same thing applies for the *yin*. *Yin* and *yang wei mai* are responsible for that. This is the reason why there are many expressions with the character *wei*.

Li Shizhen calls them 'the *gang wei* (綱 維) for the body'. *Gang* (綱) is the great principle for something, the main rope of the net. And this is one way of saying that the *wei* ensure the fundamental equilibrium in the body, through their influence on all the *yang* and all the *yin*. This is the reason why commentators have said that the *yang wei mai* masters the exterior, and the movement towards the exterior, and the *yin wei* masters the interior and the movement towards the interior.

Other texts say that *yang wei mai* has a special influence in over the defensive *qi* (*wei qi* 衛 氣) and the *yin wei mai* over the nutrition (*ying qi* 營 氣). Another text, which is quite modern, says that the meaning is to ensure all the connections of the *yang* and to ensure all the connections of the *yin*. Here the phrase *wei xi* (維 系) is used, to suggest the ability to catch both the smallest and the largest aspects. It suggests a kind of fishing net which, if it is both solid enough and fine enough, can catch every kind of fish, little fish as well as big fish. It is firm and solid and the principles unite and solidify for the greatest *yang* and the most minute *yin*. It gives the idea of connection and relationship too. We will see that many of the points given for the *wei* treat this function of the *yang* within itself and the *yin* within itself.

There is a very nice sentence in the Chinese which says:

> 'That which moves and circulates between all the *yin* meridians is called *yin wei*. That which moves and circulates between all the *yang* meridians is called *yang wei*.'

Another character used to explain *wei* is *chi* (持) which is made with a hand pointing firmly, and which means to hold and maintain.

PATHWAYS OF YIN AND YANG WEI MAI

Nanjing difficulty 28:

> '*Yang wei* and *yin wei* fasten and hold the body together (*wei luo* 維 絡) in situations of overflowing or of accumulation (*yi xu* 溢 畜) which prevent the circular movement by which irrigation is poured out to all the meridians. Thus the *yang wei* arise at the gathering of all the *yang* (*zhu yang zhi hui* 諸 陽 之 會), and the *yin wei* at the crossing of all the *yin* (*zhu yin zhi jiao* 諸 陰 之 交).'

This text gives us one of the best and most concise descriptions of the pathways of the extraordinary meridians. The first point here is that there is no pathway given for the *yin* or *yang wei mai*. They appear together and not in a separate presentation as was the case for the six other meridians. They have a common function, to fasten and hold the body together. They maintain the relationship of the *yin* and *yang* inside the body so that all the *yin* and all the *yang* are in a good relationship and in proportion.

It seems that the function is more important than the pathway here, and there is the idea that they are present everywhere. It is difficult to construct a special pathway for the *wei mai* and especially for the *yang wei mai*, as there are points given here and there in different texts, but they do not make a pathway. In the Nanjing there is no pathway given, but just this function, to fasten and hold.

The passage 'in situations of overflowing or of accumulation which prevent the circular movement by which irrigation is poured out to all the meridians' is perhaps an interpolation from another part of the text, as it is very similar to the text of difficulty 27. We cannot be sure whether it is deliberately linked here with the *wei mai*. The *wei mai* hold in order and keep everything at a good level, a bit like a water level. If the *yin* is too strong, it can prevent the *yang* circulating well. If the *yang* is too strong it can prevent the *yin* movement occurring normally, which gives rise to all kinds of blockage and lack of communication between *yin* and *yang*.

The location of the starting points for these two meridians are also given in a strange way. They are not exactly points and not exactly anatomical positions. We have these two different expressions: *zhu yin zhi jiao* (諸 陰 之 交) and *zhu yang zhi hui* (諸 陽 之 會). The meaning of *zhu* (諸) is all. And there is a variation in the last characters between *jiao* (交) and *hui* (會). *Jiao* is a meeting and a crossing. *Hui* is also a meeting, but not in the same way; it is a meeting where people gather together, an official meeting, an association, official business in a society, whereas *jiao* is more personal, relational, and includes sexual relationship. But both are a way to meet, and one is for the *yang* and the other for the *yin*; they each have their own particular way and movement. What is natural for the *yin* is this kind of intimate crossing and exchange, and the movement of gathering natural to the *yang* is more to organize in a meeting together.

This *hui* character appears in the names of seven points, and apart from the first point of the *ren mai, hui yin* (會 陰) which, as we have seen, it always has this ambivalence of *yin* and *yang,* being the meeting point of *du mai* and *ren mai.* All the others are on *yang* meridians, for example, *bai hui* (百 會 Du 20), and *hui yang* (會 陽 Bl 35). The others are all on the *shao yang* meridians, *hui zong* (會 宗 TH 7), *nao hui* (臑 會 TH 13), *ting hui* (聽 會 Gb 2) and *di wu hui* (地 五 會 Gb 42).

Conversely, we find *jiao* in *san yin jiao* (三 陰 交 Sp 6), the point for the crossing and exchange of the three *yin*, and also in *yin jiao* (陰 交 Ren 7) the general crossing and exchange of *yin*. Another point is *jiao xin* (交 信 Ki 8) which is the approach to the meeting at *san yin jiao.* Apart from that this *jiao* character can also be found in the name of *yang jiao* (陽 交 Gb 35) and finally the last point of the *du mai* (*yin jiao* 齗 交), which is the meeting point with the *ren mai*, giving a parallel with *hui yin* at the beginning of the *ren mai*, and indicating this kind of circle between *ren mai* and *du mai.*

So we can see that *jiao* is used more for the *yin*, and *hui* for the *yang*, with all the possibility of opening to exchange, through Gallbladder 35 for example, or through the first point of *ren mai* and the last point of *du mai*. And this really expresses the difference in the idea of meeting for the *yin* and the *yang*; the *yin* being most personal and internal, the *yang* more exterior. Both are equally important.

We know that both the *ren mai* and the *du mai* are present at *hui yin* (會 陰 Ren 1), and in many texts this point is given as the supporting point for the *du mai*. *Yin jiao* (斷 交 Du 28) is the junction of the *ren mai* and *du mai* in the upper body at the mouth.

Generally, these two expressions 'crossing of all the *yin*' and 'gathering of all the *yang*' are used to designate the points Kidney 9 (*zhu bin*) and Bladder 63 (*jin men*), but they are not exactly the names for these points. Other texts say that *yin wei* arises at the point Kidney 9, and the *yang wei mai* at Bladder 63. But in the Nanjing these two expressions are certainly mentioned without any indication of a pathway. It is appropriate for the *yin wei mai* to ensure all kinds of meetings and exchanges between the *yin*, and it is the main function and definition of the *yang wei mai* to be able to ensure and to rule the meeting and gathering of all the *yang*. The pathway is not the issue.

Whereas the two *qiao mai* started at exactly the same level and at the same place, the middle of the heel, here the level is quite different, because Bladder 63 is at ground level, just after the point *shen mai* (Bl 62) and for the *yin wei mai* Kidney 9 is higher.

We can see that in the description of the pathway by Li Shizhen *yin wei* rises to the top of the head by. The *yin qiao mai* merges with the *yang qiao mai* at the eyes and the brain, but the *yin wei mai* is more isolated. The *yin* and *yang wei mai* do not meet or merge with each other. Even in the pathway described by Li Shizhen, they remain quite separate. And it is by the maintenance of this difference and distinction that they are able to ensure equilibrium and a good relationship between *yin* and *yang*. If the *yang* have a good relationship amongst themselves, and the *yin* too, then the *yin* and the *yang* are automatically in a good relationship.

Li Shizhen:

'The *yin wei* (陰 維) surges from where all the *yin* make contact, *zhu yin zhi jiao* (諸 陰 之 交). Its *mai* is launched (*fa* 發) from the point *zhu bin* (築 賓 Ki 9) on the *shao yin* of the foot, which is, for the *yin wei*, a reserve (*xi* cleft point). This point is located five *cun* above the internal malleolus, in the centre where the flesh of the calf separates. The *mai* rises, running over the anterior, internal face of the thigh, and in rising, penetrates the lower abdomen. It meets with the *tai yin*, *jue yin*, *shao yin* and *yang ming* of the foot (spleen, liver, kidney and stomach meridians) at *fu she* (府 舍 Sp 13). It rises to meet *tai yin* at *da heng* (大 橫 Sp 15) and *fu ai* (腹 哀 Sp 16). It runs over the ribs and meets the *jue yin* of the foot at *qi men* (期 門 Liv 14). It rises to the thorax and diaphragm and surrounds the pharynx. It meets with *ren mai* at *tian tu* (天 突 Ren 22) and *lian quan* (廉 泉 Ren 23), and rises to reach the front of the top of the head where it ends. In all 14 points.

The *yang wei* (陽 維) surges from the meeting of all the
yang, zhu yang zhi hui (諸 陽 之 會). Its *mai* is launched (*fa*
發) from the point *jin men* (金 門 Bl 63) of the *tai yang* of
the foot, which is located on the foot, one and a half *cun*
below the external malleolus. It rises to seven *cun* above
the malleolus where it meets the *shao yang* of the foot at
yang jiao (陽 交 Gb 35) which is its reserve (*xi* cleft point).
It runs over the knee on the external face and rising by
the depression along the femur, reaches the side of the
lower abdomen. It meets with the *shao yang* of the foot at
ju liao (Gb 29). It runs over the ribs, rising obliquely over
them; it meets the *yang ming* of the hand (large intestine
meridian) and *tai yang* of the foot and hand (bladder and
small intestine meridians) at *bi nao* (臂 臑 LI 14); it passes
to the front of the shoulder and meets the *shao yang* of
the hand (triple heater meridian) at *nao hui* (臑 會 TH
13) and *jian liao* (TH 15). It returns and meets the *shao
yang* of the foot and hand and the *yang ming* of the foot
(gallbladder, triple heater and stomach meridians) at *jian
jing* (肩 井 GB 21).

It penetrates behind the shoulder and meets the *tai
yang* of the hand (small intestine meridian) and the *yang
qiao* at *nao yu* (臑 俞 SI 10). It rises and runs along the
back of the ear; it meets the *shao yang* of the hand and
foot (triple heater and gallbladder) at *feng chi* (風 池 Gb
20); it rises to *nao kong* (腦 空 Gb 19), *cheng ling* (承 靈
Gb 18), *zheng ying* (正 營 Gb 17), *mu chuang* (目 窗 Gb 16)
and *lin qi* (臨 泣 Gb 15). It descends onto the forehead and

creates a meeting with the five *mai*: *shao yang* of the foot and hand (gallbladder and triple heater meridians), *yang ming* of the foot and hand (stomach and large intestine meridians) at *yang bai* (陽 白 Gb 14). It runs along the head and penetrates the ear. It rises to *ben shen* (本 神 Gb 13) and stops. In all 32 points.'

The pathway of *yin wei mai* includes the points Kidney 9, Spleen 13, 15, 16, Liver 14 and Ren 22 and 23. Spleen 12 is often mentioned in association with the *yin wei mai* but it is not in the pathway given by Li Shizhen. The three *yin* of the foot, kidney, spleen and liver, and the *ren mai* are represented, which is a way to suggest this kind of meeting of the *yin* power.

It is the same for the *yang wei*. Here are all the points found in Li Shizhen and different classical texts: Bladder 63, Gallbladder 35, 29, 24, Large Intestine 14, Triple Heater 13,15, Small Intestine 10, Du 15, 16, Stomach 1 and Gallbladder 13 - 21. There are 20 points, but they are never given all together. The most I have found is 18 points, but there are many differences in presentation of the *yang wei*. Sometimes it reaches the top of the head by the forehead, other times by the nape of the neck, it is difficult to find consistency and make one definitive pathway for the *yang wei mai*. And perhaps it is not necessary.

All the *yang* meridians are represented here, the gallbladder being the most strongly indicated. This pathway is almost a symbolic way to assert that the *yang wei mai* supports each quality of *yang qi* and each expression of the *yang*. We can see the *yang wei* like a constellation present in the *yang* and behind the *yang* movement, and you can touch these functions with these points on each *yang* meridian.

Claude Larre: The description of life and the function of life are quite different. For the description we have to differentiate between one point and another, for the functioning of life all those distinctions disappear, because the functioning of life merges with other functions. But our analytical mind is not prepared to receive that sort of information because it is contrary to our habits. So whenever we feel that it is difficult to understand, it is not that the explanation is difficult to understand, it is because we are asking things in our mind which are not really the way life is. We have the representation of the unity of life, and at that very moment we are given a description of so many scattered things. Then we do not understand. Or we are interested by the scattering and then the necessity of the unity of life comes into the mind. So 99% of the difficulty comes from the way we are managing our mind in relationship with text. It is only time which makes it flow and merge one with the other.

Elisabeth Rochat: In Li Shizhen's description, the *yang wei mai* follows the gallbladder meridian and crosses the head from back to front. But in some other texts we can find the opposite movement, from front to back. In this case the *yang wei mai* finishes at Du 15 and 16. This is interesting because it reflects the end of the *yin wei mai* at Ren 22 and 23. These last two extraordinary meridians, responsible for the *yin* and the *yang* merge into the two most primitive meridians responsible at the origin for the *yin* and the *yang*.

I think I prefer this presentation because it closes the circle very nicely.

Now we can see that the *wei mai*, which are responsible for the maintenance of organization and order within the *yang* and the *yin*, have to rely on the *ren mai* and *du mai*, and also connect to the other meridians. A pathway or description of a trajectory is a way to indicate the quality of the *qi* and the function, and the place where this function can be rooted. Maybe there is no pathway, just an image, because the most important thing is the function that the pathway symbolizes. We must not limit the effect of a meridian just to a line; in the same way that we do not limit the effect of a *zang* or *fu* to the anatomical mass.

Question: Why is a special emphasis given to the *xi* cleft points in the text?

Elisabeth Rochat: At *yang jiao* (陽 交 Gb 35) there is a particular reserve for the *yang wei mai*, and the meaning is that in this place you can touch a certain quality of *qi* and create a certain vital movement in the patient which is in touch with the function of the *yang wei mai*. It is perhaps not by chance that this character *jiao* is the same character we found in the anchorage point for the *yin wei mai*. We do not know the limit of our imagination and perhaps we do not know the limit of all the Chinese speculations, but we must pay attention to whether these speculations were the thought of just one person, or whether they were general enough to be part of the culture.

PATHOLOGY OF YIN AND YANG WEI MAI

Nanjing difficulty 29:

> 'When the extraordinary meridians give rise to illnesses what are they like?

> 'Well, *yang wei* connects the *yang*, *yin wei* connects the *yin*. If *yin* and *yang* cannot connect with one another then there is vexation (*chang ran* 恨 然) and loss of will (*shi zhi* 失 志). One is without strength, and one no longer has a hold on oneself.

> 'When *yang wei* gives rise to illnesses one suffers from cold and heat. When *yin wei* gives rise to illnesses one suffers pains in the heart.'

Elisabeth Rochat: The first description gives a pathology for both *yin* and *yang wei mai*, without differentiation. The *wei* function is unable to ensure the relationship between *yin* and *yang* and there is deep dejection and a loss of will. This is the loss of the power to maintain and hold the very central principle of the direction of life, the movement of *qi*, the will. The heart is completely dejected and is unable to find the joy of the spirit and a good circulation of life. Loss of will is the loss of the stability and solidity of the base that life depends on. That is the result of the lack of the *wei* function on the *yin* and *yang* everywhere in the body. One is without strength, and no longer has a hold on oneself.

The Chinese character to hold (*chi* 抶) is often used to

202 • THE EIGHT EXTRAORDINARY MERIDIANS

explain the *wei* function. What are we are unable to hold? Everything! We are unable to hold an idea. We are unable to maintain purpose or intent, unable to hold anything in the hand, because the *yang* is too weak and there is a scattering of the muscular strength and all the connections between bones and flesh and muscles. And the heart is not in a good state. This is a very general condition; everything unravels, there is a mental state of dejection and a loss of connection between the heart and kidneys. It is also the inability to hold onto one's true nature.

After that there is a presentation of the symptoms appropriate to the *yang wei mai*, and symptoms appropriate to the *yin wei mai*, and they are completely different. In the case of the *qiao mai* the symptoms presented for the *yang* and the *yin qiao mai* were very often parallel, possibly the contrary of each other, for example if the *yin* is tense, the *yang* is loose. Or there is a play between insomnia and sleepiness – very often the symptoms are simply opposites. But here in the case of the *wei mai* the symptoms are completely different. There is no connection between the symptoms of cold and heat and pain in the heart. That is another way to emphasize the difference between the *yin* and the *yang*.

So what is this cold and heat? It is the inability of the defensive *qi* to protect against exterior influences and perverse influences, and this is linked with the *yang wei mai* which is responsible for the exterior, responsible for the *yang* and especially for defence. If the firmness and solidity, which must be maintained at the exterior of the body by the *yang qi*, is too weak, it is a pathology of the *yang wei mai.* One of the main symptoms will be fear of the cold, and cold with fever. There is over-sensitivity to cold and heat and also, perhaps for the first time in the pathology of the eight extraordinary meridians, a very strong relationship with perverse energy coming from the exterior. Remember that the four attachments (*si wei* 四 維) also suggest the four limbs, and the four limbs are said to be the place of the defensive *qi* – especially the extremities, which could be described as our own four attachments to the exterior.

The strong relationship between the *yang wei mai* and the gallbladder meridian, the *shao yang* of the foot, reminds us of the quality of *shao yang* to be the pivot, and this pathology of cold and heat is the same as the intermittent fevers often linked with the pathology of *shao yang.*

'When *yin wei* gives rise to illness one suffers pains in the heart.'

The pathology of *yin wei mai* is concerned with the *zang,* particularly the *zang* of the innermost part of the body which is in charge of the blood, the heart. This is the meaning of this symptom. Pain in the heart can be linked with the *yin wei,* but it is also a way to symbolize that the *yin wei* is linked to the blood, to the nutrition and to the internal part, the *li* (理), and the best way to sum that up is the symptom of pain in the heart.

The general symptom for *yin* and *yang* is a kind of general loosening at each level, but if we want to specify the *yang wei* and the *yin wei,* there is a symptom which emphasizes the *yang* activity and the *yang* responsibility of the *yang wei mai* at the exterior of the body with the defensive *qi*, and for the *yin* the contrary.

The symptoms of cold and heat suggest all the possible pathology of the *yang*; the deficiency of the *yang* in defence, and a kind of exaggeration of the *yang* sometimes due to a deficiency or perverse *qi* leading to fever. In the case of the symptoms of *yin wei mai*, this pain in the heart suggests all kinds of possible obstruction in the chest and thorax, possibly due to the action of the cold, which is an exaggeration of the *yin* movement and the *yin* quality. There may be obstruction of the circulation especially in the spleen and kidney meridians, which have very close relationships with *yin wei mai*; the kidney meridian being the starting point of *yin wei mai*, and the spleen having several points in common. There may also be all kinds of counter-current in the liver meridian or *ren mai*. That is all represented by the points given to the *yin wei mai*.

There are no special symptoms given to the *wei mai* in other texts, only variations on this same pathology.

SUMMARY OF THE WEI MAI

Elisabeth Rochat: *Chong mai* provides a unity of the *yin* and *yang*, the sea of blood and the sea of meridians. It is the starting point for all the crossing of *yin* and *yang* and occupies all the space of the form of the body. With the *wei mai* there is also this kind of differentiation and organization of the system, the *yang* system and the *yin* system. The *zang* and the *fu*, the *yang* meridians and the *yin* meridians, the defence and the nutrition, the *biao* and the *li* must all be maintained in good relationship with the other pathways, the *yin* meridians with the *yang* meridians (especially the coupled ones) the *zang* with the *fu*, the interior with the exterior; the defence with the nutrition and the *qi* with the blood. This is an expression of the *wei mai*, and a kind of link made with *chong mai* and *dai mai*.

The relationship between the *qiao mai* and *ren mai* and *du mai* is at the level of the rising spring of life, with a merging one into the other. The *ren mai* and *du mai* merge into one another as do the *qiao mai*.

With the *chong mai* and *dai mai* there is a different movement, and it is the same with the *wei mai*. Each commands their own territory and system – but in order to allow communication and balance between them, because one cannot exist without the other. This is always the basic premise. They express all kinds of basic relationships within the *yin* and the *yang* systems. Perhaps they also represent, with this idea of the four attachments and the four limbs and the four directions, the complete extension of the body. Their two particular points are on the heart master (pericardium) meridian, *nei guan* (內 關 P 6) and on the triple heater meridian, *wai guan* (外 關 TH 5). The names of these points also express this. Both point names contain the same character *guan* (關) and both are the *luo* points of the heart master and triple heater meridians. One is turned to the interior (*nei* 內) the other to the exterior (*wai* 外). The parallelism between these two points is quite evident.

Nei guan (P 6) has a special relationship with the *zang* and the interior, and with the pathology of congestion and obstruction of the heart and the thorax. For instance, the hampering of circulation of blood and nutrition, coming from the heart and the chest.

Wai guan (TH 5) is a point to restore all kinds of circulation, the two points making a kind of double passage for circulation. *Guan* is a pass, a place where there is a passage – but it is under control. This is a kind of double articulation, because *guan* can also have the meaning of articulation, to the inside or to the outside in this kind of paired position on the arm. Both being *luo* points, *wai guan* is in a *luo* relationship with the heart master meridian and *nei guan* with the triple heater meridian, to ensure the equilibrium between one and the other.

If we refer to the pathology of the *wei mai*, *nei guan* is a very good point to treat the kind of pain in the heart linked with the *yin wei mai*. And *wai guan*, as a point on the *shao yang* meridian, is a perfect point to treat cold and heat from the exterior. The defensive *qi* is linked with the ability of the triple heater to distribute the *qi* – the middle heater to assimilate enough essences coming from food, the lower heater to give these influences the *yang* forces of defence, and the ability of the upper heater to make them circulate well. So these two points are particularly well chosen for the pathology of the *wei mai*, and they are related by their position, by their function, and by their names.

The expression *nei guan* is found in the Lingshu, not as a point name, but as a pathological situation of blockage, when the *yin* and the *yang* are no longer communicating well. The *yang* is blocked at the exterior and the *yin* blocked in the interior and there a lack of communication between these two systems. This point *nei guan* is also used when the *yin* is blocked in the interior and the *yang* is unable to penetrate the *yin* and restore the balance between the two. All these kinds of connections are between the *biao* and the *li*, the *yang wei mai* mastering the *biao* and the *yin wei mai* the *li*.

The pathology of the *qiao mai* was more internal. In insomnia and somnolence there is more concern with biorhythms than the relationship with the exterior. The *yang wei mai* have the pathology of cold and heat and a relationship with the exterior and the *qi* coming from external influences, which change everyday. For the *yang* and *yin qiao mai* it was rather the adaptation of our own biorhythm to the rhythm of the universe, and the normal succession of *yin* and *yang*.

Question: Could you say a little more on the difference between *men* (門) and *guan* (關)?

Elisabeth Rochat: *Men* (門) is a great opening of something. The character *guan* (關) has the same opening, but with something inside to control what is passing through. I think that is the main difference.

Claude Larre: *Guan* is used for the customs in the harbour. You may pass through but you have to stop. And it can be closed. If you pay the correct tax you can pass through. It is often used in China to pass from one place to another, a kind of frontier control or barrier, often involving the payment of a toll. *Guan* can also be a pass in the mountain, more than simply a wall with a door.

Elisabeth Rochat: This character *guan* can mean to put into communication and to keep in touch, as well as to close something, and to separate.

Question: Could you say something about the paired meridians which share the same master and coupled points?

Elisabeth Rochat: It is really a question of the area of the body which is concerned. For instance, *du mai* and *yang qiao mai* are associated with the points *hou xi*, Small Intestine 3, and *shen mai*, Bladder 62. The indications are for abnormalities occurring at the inner corner of the eyes, the nape of the neck, the shoulder and all that. It is a way to treat the *yang* in its greatest extension through the *tai yang* meridian. And it is related to the *du mai* and the *yang qiao mai* through the effect of rising the *yang* to supply the *yang* areas of the body and especially the upper part of the body, the top of the body and the top of the back.

For the *chong mai* and *yin wei mai*, *gong sun*, Spleen 4, and *nei guan*, Heart Master (Pericardium) 6, treat all kinds of perturbation and stagnation of the chest and the heart and the middle heater. And it is the conjunction of these two points that is used to free the area of the upper heater and middle heater of congestion.

Dai mai and *yang wei mai* are associated with *lin qi*, Gallbladder 41, and *wai guan*, Triple Heater 5, which affect the lateral part of the upper body, not so central as the *du mai* and *yang qiao mai*. The main areas are the external corner of the eyes, the back of the ear, and the cheeks and shoulders but in a lateral view.

With *lie que*, Lung 7, and *zhao hai*, Kidney 6, there is the whole system of the diaphragm, the functioning of the lungs and the chest through the throat and pharynx. And this is the difference, for instance, between *yin wei mai* and *chong mai*, where the effect was rather below the diaphragm. The end of the pathway of the kidney meridian goes up through the throat to the root of the tongue, and there is an ascending movement accompanying the *ren mai*, and the ascending movement of the *yin* inside the body. We can use these two points for that.

We can see an aspect of the general function of the extraordinary meridians in these points, and also where these particular functions may be treated. For example, the *chong mai* has a relationship with the stomach and the spleen, and the middle heater, and also with the heart. The *yin wei mai* has something to do with the inner *zang* and especially with the heart through the blood, the nutrition and so on. These two points are very well chosen to free this area, and in freeing this area to help the restoration of the functions which are under the authority of these extraordinary meridians.

It is the same thing for the *du mai* and the *yang qiao mai*, and the *dai mai* and the *yang wei mai*, to be more exterior, lateral and enveloping. If there is the ability to make volume, there is also the ability with the gallbladder meridian to create a laterality. The gallbladder meridian has an important role and presence within the extraordinary meridians.

Question: Are the terms 'master and couple point' translations of the Chinese?

Elisabeth Rochat: In the Zhenjiu Dacheng, The Great Compendium of Acupuncture and Moxibustion, the points *gong sun*, Spleen 4, and *nei guan*, Heart Master 6, are said to be 'in free circulation with the *chong mai*', and 'in free circulation with the *yin wei mai*'. After that they say that there is a conjunction of the effect of these two points at the heart, thorax and stomach. And the sentence construction is the same for the others. This is not the first book to present this kind of systematisation of the eight meridians. There are other presentations of the coupling of these points which say that they are in resonance with each other and with the eight extraordinary meridians.

CONCLUSION

Elisabeth Rochat: I do not think that we need to make a résumé of the whole construction of the eight extraordinary meridians because we have repeated it many times. There are many personal visions and particular theories belonging to certain schools, they are all very interesting in practice but each has the perspective of an individual school.

The eight extraordinary meridians are important in daoist meditation and visualisation because they provide a way to retrieve and imagine the first organization of life and the dynamism of the process of this organization – from the state of unity, the first beginnings, through to the completely achieved body. We can understand how the daoist adepts worked on these meridians to put the circulation and *yin* and *yang* in order at each level, to discover their origin and to find their unity in the process of their continuing lives. There are many ways of working with the eight extraordinary meridians within the body using visualisation and internal exercises for the *qi* and the breath.

'Human beings possess these eight meridians, they all belong to the *yin* and the spirits. The sage is able to reach the *dao* by the way of these eight meridians. These eight meridians are the root of the great way of pre-heaven, and ancestor of the one unique *qi*.'

This is an extract from a daoist text which explains the value of the inner alchemy of the eight extraordinary meridians as the root and beginning of all things, particularly the concentration and distribution of authentic *qi*. The daoist vision, for example in Zhuangzi, is the possibility of concentrating the *qi* in a kind of cohesion of all the manifestations that *qi* can take. The diffusion of *qi* is scattering, separation and death, but it is at the same time movement and preservation of the equilibrium. If these eight *mai* are really representative of that, then they provide the daoist adept a good way to work inside the body. But these particular techniques are not a part of the medical texts. The daoist alchemical teachings are a way to understand life, and the processes of life. They may be useful in treatment, but they are not exactly the same thing.

Claude Larre: These texts, whether medical or daoist, were not written from our point of view. The authors were quite possibly writing from their own experience, and writing from experience is writing from their way of being one with life. We must attempt to understand life by the way it moves and by the way in which it appears. Being practitioners we have a better opportunity to understand, because what is taught may be true at the level of teaching, but not necessarily at the level of experience. And if we are not able to make the distinction between the teaching and the experience then we are lost.

All Chinese texts consider the unknown, the invisible, that which is alluded to or not. That is one of the less understood aspects of all the texts. A large part of divination, which is to see through the invisible, requires that we first have experience of life. We are experimenting with our own life and the life of the patient reciprocally. And there lies the mystery, the difficulty and the danger.

INDEX

INDEX

THE TEXTS:

Translation of the texts of the Neijing Suwen and Lingshu were
made by Claude Larre and Elisabeth Rochat de la Vallée over
a number of years from a number of sources, but particular
reference has been made to the following:

古今圖書集成　醫部全錄
人民衛生出版社
Beijing 1959

素 問注釋匯粹
人民衛生出版社
Beijing 1982